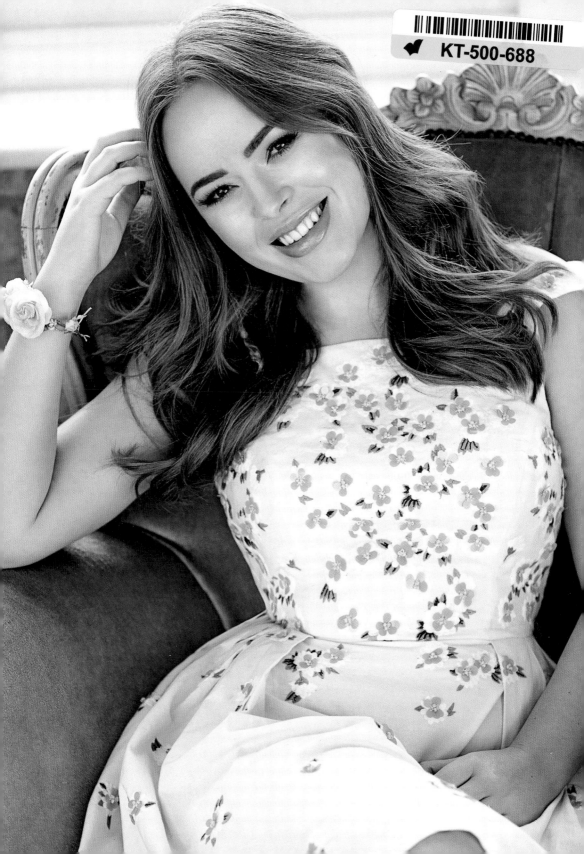

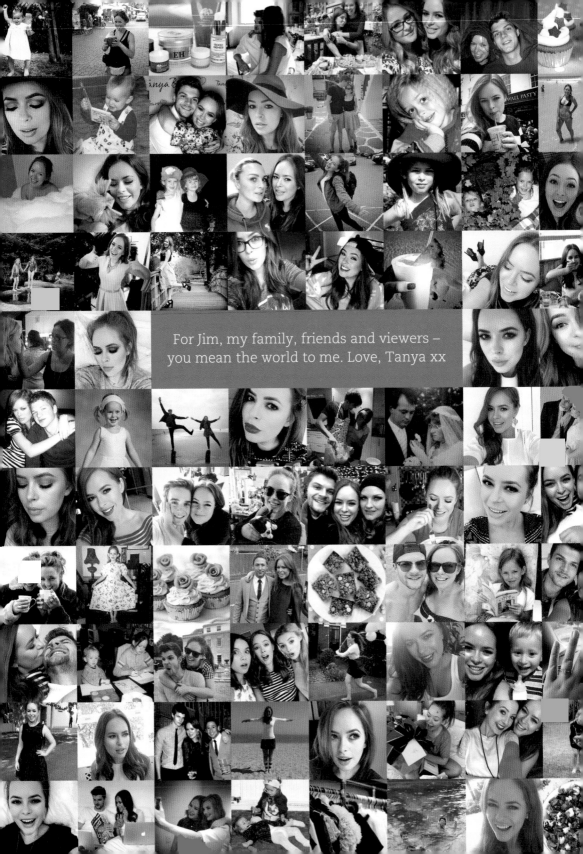

For Jim, my family, friends and viewers – you mean the world to me. Love, Tanya xx

LOVE
TANYA

MICHAEL JOSEPH
an imprint of
PENGUIN BOOKS

With thanks to the following stockists for the photoshoot outfits:
1) Long nude floral embellished dress – Yuvna Kim. 2) Black shorts – River Island; white T-shirt – French Connection; necklaces – Jennifer Zeuner and Kasun London; black bra – Freya. 3) Floral dress – French Connection. 4) Black bodysuit – Oh My Love; cowgirl jacket – Rokit; black hat – Topshop. 5) Long cream skirt – Nevena; grey T-shirt – River Island. 6) Gold dress – Prey of London; sequin jacket – Vintage; boots – Dune. 7) Sequin top – Zara. 8) Lips top – Oasis. 9) Fake feather jacket – Topshop; leather leggings – Richard Radcliffe; shoes – Sergio Rossi. 10) Pink jumper – Zara. 11) Black-and-white column dress – Roland Mouret; black tuxedo jacket – Reiss. 12) Vest – Aloe.

Quotation on p.152 from *Modern Family*, season three, episode nine (written by Steven Levitan, Christopher Lloyd and Ben Karlin).

Every effort has been made to contact copyright holders. The publishers will be glad to correct any errors or omissions in future editions.

MICHAEL JOSEPH

UK | USA | Canada | Ireland | Australia
India | New Zealand | South Africa

Michael Joseph is part of the Penguin Random House group of companies whose addresses can be found at global.penguinrandomhouse.com.

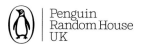

Penguin
Random House
UK

First published 2015
005

All photographs by Dan Kennedy, Matt Russell and Tanya Burr
with the exception of those appearing courtesy of the following:
Getty: pp.7, 127, 133, 134, 149, 245, 252, 290, 291. Shutterstock: pp.131, 209
Craig Fordham: pp.125, 268, 271

Designed and set in 10.5/16pt PMN Caecilia by Smith & Gilmour
Colour reproduction by Altaimage, London
Printed and bound in Italy by L.E.G.O. S.p.A.

A CIP catalogue record for this book is available from the British Library

ISBN: 978-1-405-92140-4

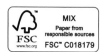

CONTENTS

PROLOGUE

As we drew up beside the pavement in front of the Sanderson Hotel, light bulbs started flashing before I had even opened the door of the car. I felt sick with nerves but at the same time, I was really excited and couldn't wait to go inside.

Jim gave my hand a squeeze. 'Ready?' he asked.

I took a deep breath and stepped out onto the street. One of my biggest fears was that no one at all would turn up and I certainly hadn't expected there to be photographers waiting for me. It all felt really surreal. It was 30th January 2014 and the launch night of Tanya Burr Cosmetics. I had been working on the range for more than eighteen months and really wanted everyone to love the products as much as I did. This party felt like the culmination of many, many hours of meetings, designing and hard work.

Entering the party, I just couldn't believe how many friendly faces were there. My best friends from home like Maddie, Vanessa, Kate and Emma were there to support me, along with YouTube friends such as Zoe, Joe and Alfie and, of course, my amazingly supportive family – Mum, Dad, little sister Tasha and little brother Oscar, and my fiancée Jim. Everyone was enjoying the cocktails, and yummy canapés and looking around, I felt a buzz of happiness and excitement. All of the finished products were displayed and lit up on surfaces around the venue and looked amazing.

The evening went past in a blur and when it got to 10 p.m. and the launch was supposed to be winding up, it seemed busier than ever, but I figured by that point, it would be OK to sneak away. A lovely man at the hotel organised for me to get a private room with twenty of my closest friends and family so I could spend some quality time with them, as during the party I had been doing interview after interview with lots of different journalists. The man led us into this cute little room with a table inside, just big enough for us all to squeeze round and grab some food. As it was quite late, instead of a proper dinner we had all the Crème Egg brownies that my friend Scarlett had made me. Looking around, all the people I loved in one place, it just felt incredible. Everyone was so supportive and that meant the world to me.

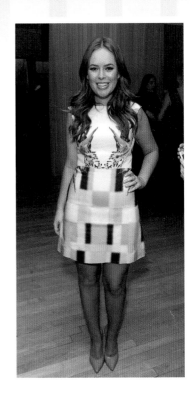

This launch is just one of the many amazing things that has happened to me since I started making videos and uploading them to YouTube back in 2009. I feel like I need to pinch myself to see if it's really real, and it makes me feel really choked up just thinking about it. I often have these moments, where I sit back and I think, 'This is just insane.' It just reminds me just how lucky I am and how far I have come in such a short time.

Thanks for picking up my book! I'm so excited to be writing it, for loads of different reasons. I hope to give you more of an insight into my childhood and life growing up in Norfolk, tell you about why I started making videos and the journey I have been on since: full of fun, surprises, meeting some wonderful people, getting engaged to Jim, moving to London and launching my cosmetics line.

I also want to give you all some practical beauty, style and lifestyle tips and help you feel more confident. I always try to be happy and upbeat, but as any girl knows, growing up – and being a grown-up – isn't always easy and I hope to show you some of the tricks and tips I use to help me feel self-assured.

As some of you might know, I have also suffered from anxiety and panic attacks and I will tell you more about how I have learned to deal with this in the hope it will help any of you affected by similar issues. I will talk about my friendships and relationships and all the everyday stuff that goes on behind my videos. I've also left space for you to add your own scrapbook-style lists, so you can jot down different ideas about what you want to achieve, ways you can feel happier, things you want to explore online or places you want to see. I really want you to get involved, so grab your pen and get writing!

Finally, I just wanted to say thank you. I love, love, love, what I do: writing my blog, filming my videos, working on Tanya Burr Cosmetics and always having exciting projects in the pipeline. But the best thing of all is speaking to my viewers every day. I wouldn't be doing any of this without you guys and I am so grateful for your support. I love reading all your comments and tweets and feel so lucky that I get to chat to people I think of as friends all around the world. Let me know what you think of my book – I can't wait to read your feedback. Happy reading!

Love, Tanya xx

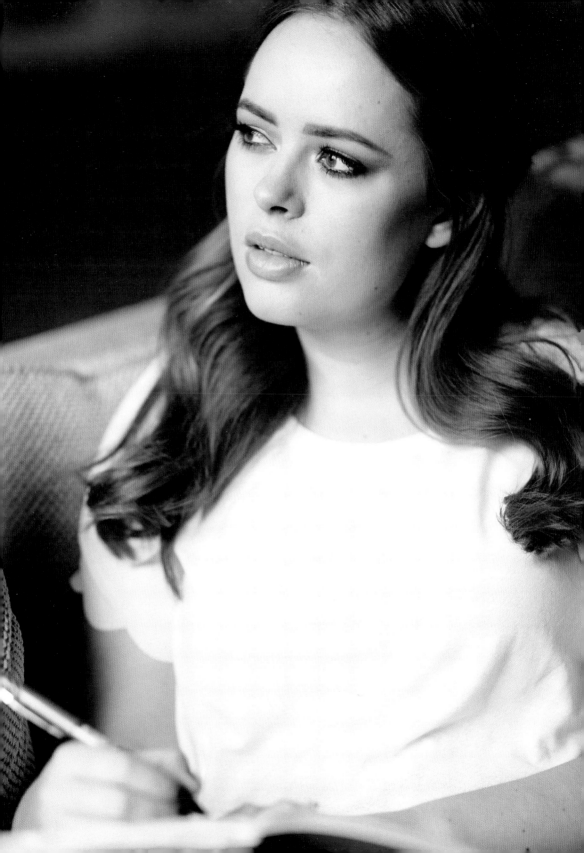

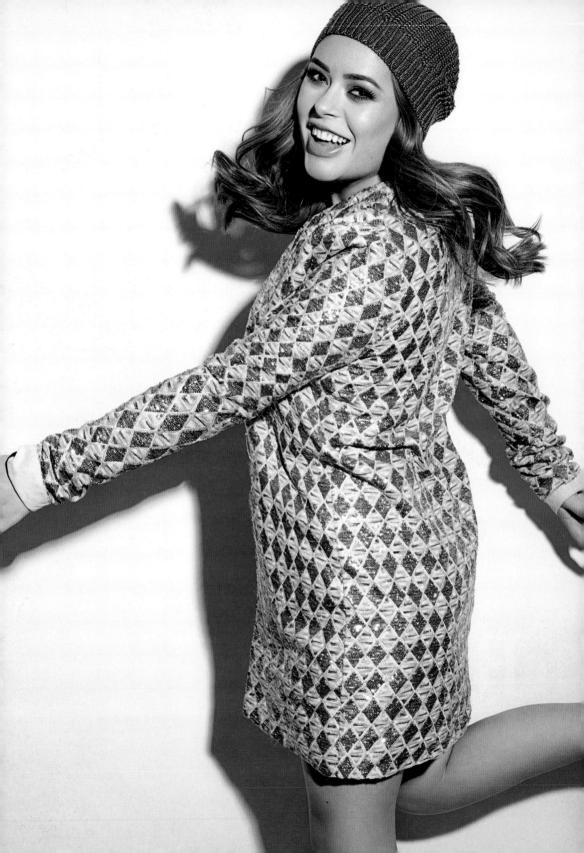

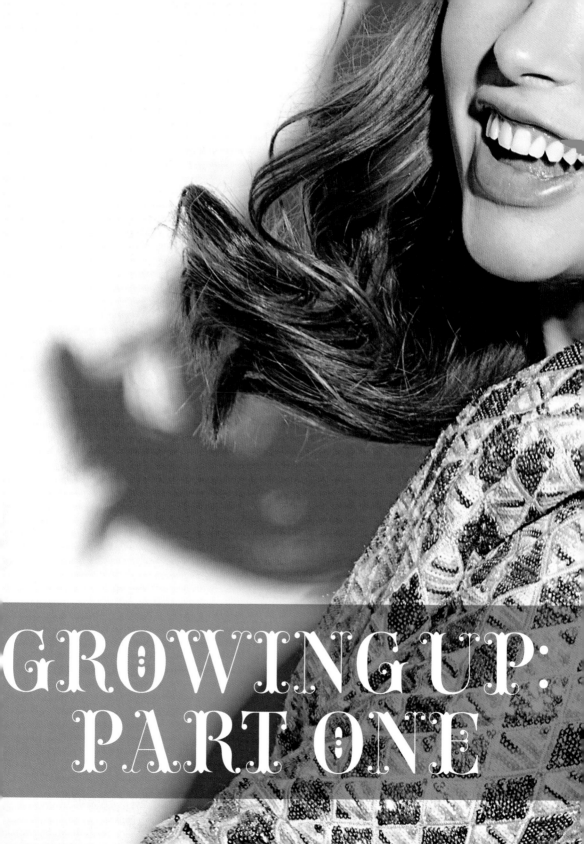

GROWING UP: PART ONE

My story started long before I was born, when Mum, whose name is Melanie, scribbled in her maths notebook, 'Mel for Neil', 'I love Neil' and their initials in love hearts one day in the classroom. She was just twelve at the time and Neil was a boy in the year above, who was one of the cool kids and was always making people laugh and being naughty. Mum was very studious and quite shy, so it wasn't an obvious match. However, they became good friends and when Mum was eighteen and Dad was nineteen, they got together and that was it; they have been together ever since. When I was little, Mum showed me the scribbles in her maths book, which she retrieved from her jewellery box, and I love the fact that she has kept it.

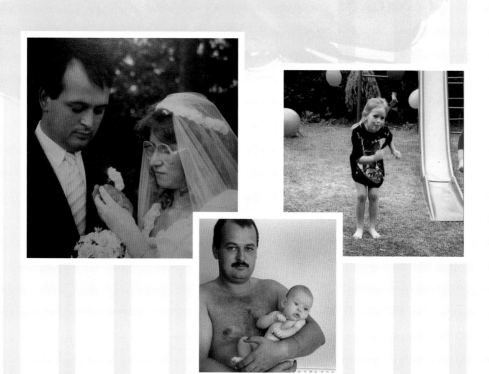

Mum and Dad bought their first home in the village of Tasburgh in Norfolk a few years later and a year after that, when they were both twenty-five, they tied the knot in a small ceremony for just their closest family and friends. Both Mum and Dad were really keen to start a family and had planned to have a baby for ages. Mum marked down the dates in her work calendar (she was working in an office at the time) and was hoping for a late spring or early summer baby. I was born on 9th June 1989.

When I was little, we would go for long walks in the countryside and down the lane nearby to a farm where there were chickens and cows and we would buy eggs, milk and cooking apples. We also went to the park, blackberry picking and to see local friends in the village. It was a real countryside upbringing. Our house was in a cul-de-sac and it was really quiet. Sometimes my old cat Casper used to fall asleep in the middle of the road and if a car came along, they would stop and pick him up and put him on the grass verge before continuing.

Dad worked long hours driving lorries for an oil company. He had been doing the job since he left school when he was sixteen and some of my happiest memories are the times when he used to come home for his lunch if he was driving in our area. I would see his enormous lorry pull up outside the house from the big window in our living room. I would always be elated to see him and rush to the door to greet him. On other occasions he would bring heating oil to our house and I remember the big pipes, his heavy boots and the strong petrol smell of the chemicals.

Dad hated his job driving lorries but has always been

really entrepreneurial and in his spare time, he used to do art classes. In our garage he had a massive lathe and he used to craft lots of wooden furniture and sell it on to make some more money. He also made loads of things in our house, like tables, chairs and lamp bases. When I was about two or three years old, apparently I used to go around saying, 'Daddy made it, Daddy made it' and point at almost every piece of furniture because I literally thought he made everything! When I was at school, he slipped a disc in his back and ended up having a year off work. In that time he studied web design and later he started his own business, which has become pretty successful. We were all really happy that he didn't have to drive lorries any more.

Two years and two days after I was born, my little sister Natasha, who we call Tash or Tasha, arrived. I loved looking after her and apparently one of my favourite things was getting her dressed and undressed — it was like she was my little dolly! I also loved helping Mum to change her nappy and do things like that. We did bicker growing up but we have always been very close. Dad would hate it if we ever argued and always made us hug and make up.

My first school was Henry Preston Primary School and it was opposite my house, so I would literally cross the road to get there and always spoke to Mum through the gate or over the hedge on my lunch break. The school was so small and friendly and I always felt happy there, even

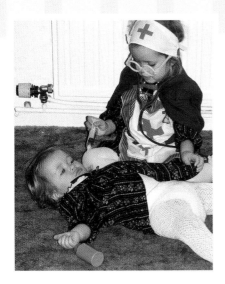
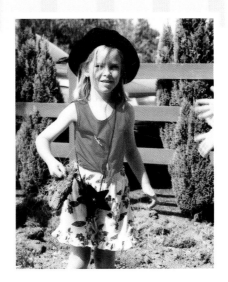

though I do remember being a bit scared of my headteacher.

My teacher in the last two years, Mrs Piggott, really left a lasting impression on me. There have been certain people in my life who have made me feel like I can do anything and she was one of them. She was a really strong woman and a bit of a hippy. She wore knitted crochet crop tops with her belly button showing, paired with floral maxi-skirts, and her hair up in a messy bun; it was a pretty cool look for a teacher, if you ask me! I took piano lessons and she taught me guitar and really encouraged my musical side. On Friday afternoons, we always sat on the floor and sung along, while she played the guitar.

I did an after-school activity every night of the week. I started ballet when I was two and then went on to do tap, jazz, disco, modern and gym. Mum and Dad wanted me to be confident and have different skills and while I don't think I was particularly good at dancing, I loved it. Mum told me that when I had a routine development check at about four years old, before starting school, the nurse asked me what a lake was and I replied, 'It's something you dance on', because I was so obsessed with the ballet, *Swan Lake*. The nurse said to Mum, 'This child is different!'

When I was small, Mum started working as a child-minder, which was really cool because it meant she was at home with us and there were always other children in the house to play with. There was one little boy she looked after whose mother was an artist and sometimes we would go to her studio half a mile down the road and have art lessons, where we made things out of clay. We never watched much television. We did have a video player, though, and I've always loved Disney. I remember we were given *Cinderella* and *Lady and the Tramp* and we watched them over and over and, later, we had *Beauty and the Beast*, which is still a real favourite of mine. Mostly though, we played with toys or outside in the garden with the other children. Mum had left school at sixteen, but alongside her child-minding work and looking after us, she went to night school to study for her A-Levels and from there, she went on to study for a degree in English Literature at the University of East Anglia (UEA) in Norwich, then she did a part-time Masters and a PGCE about a decade later. She is now an English teacher and, looking back, I think she did brilliantly bringing us up and studying at the same time. Sometimes, when Mum was studying in the evenings and I was a bit older, Dad would let us watch programmes like *EastEnders*, which Mum would never normally allow.

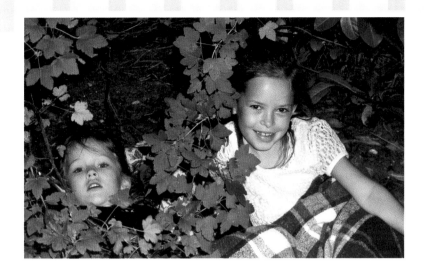

Sometimes she used to take me with her to lectures, where I learnt about literature and history from a very young age (when I managed to listen!). I would eat these enormous chocolate muffins afterwards from the university café. I asked her recently whether they were really as big as I remembered – and apparently they were!

As I got more independent, I spent most of my free time outside playing with the other children in the village. I met one of my best friends, Emma, at school. She is two years younger than me and was my sister's friend first. Me, my sister, Emma and a couple of other girls in the village would all hang out. In the summer, we made dens in the woods or we went on bike rides. We also spent loads of our time making up and performing plays. Being the oldest in the group, I ended up being the leader. I would say the words and make Emma write them down – I was quite bossy! Emma reminded me recently that I would say to her, 'You need to go home and have this typed up for our rehearsals tomorrow!' Apparently she would always spend half the night typing the script up and putting everyone's lines in different colours and the next day would bring us all printed copies. Amazing!

We spent a lot of time with my nanny and granddad, my mum's parents, who live in Newton Flotman, which is a couple of miles up the road from Tasburgh. I grew up so close to them and spent a lot of time with them before I started going to school, and when I was at school, we went to their house every Sunday for lunch. Sometimes, I would also bike to see them with my little group of friends and Nanny would always be so happy to see us and give us cartons of apple juice and something to eat before we cycled back home.

When I was eleven, I moved to the local secondary school, Long Stratton High School, which is in a different village. In primary school, there had only been twelve children in my class, so moving to a big secondary school felt scary. I don't think I have ever been so nervous. There were too many children in Tasburgh going to the school, so the main bus, which all my friends got on, was full and I was sent onto a different bus. I remember everything about that moment, like what I was wearing and how nervous I felt. I didn't know anyone and all the older kids were talking about things I didn't understand and people I didn't know. I also used to get the worst travel sickness – I still do now – and this bus went all around the windy country roads to pick up all the kids from the little villages

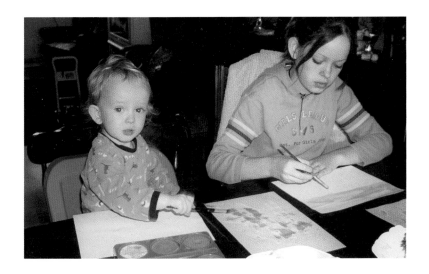

nearby. I used to feel so sick by the time I got to school. In the end, Mum managed to get me onto the main bus and I felt much happier. And eventually, of course, I settled into high school and made some good friends, Kate, who moved to Tasburgh around that time, and Maddie. I also had some really special friendships with a few other girls. Two years later, Emma and my sister joined too – so I had my little close circle of friends around me.

When I was twelve, my parents had my little brother Oscar. He was born on 3rd May 2001 and I was so thrilled. He was so adorable and the best thing ever! I used to change his nappy, dress him and play with him while Mum cooked the dinner or was busy. He was just so cute and always liked to go to sleep on someone's shoulder, so Tasha and I always cuddled him. Bathing babies is quite hard because they are so small and slippery, so if one of us was having a bath, Mum would pop him in with us. He almost felt like my baby and we all loved him so much. Mum said it was as though he had three mothers!

I got my first bout of anxiety when I was thirteen. I think I was always a slightly anxious child but this was the first time it really affected me and it seemed like it came on almost overnight. I felt so horrible and didn't even know what anxiety meant or what panic attacks were. I didn't tell anyone at first because I was scared they would think I was crazy. I had my first panic attack watching *The Terminator* and even now, if *The Terminator* comes up in conversations or on repeat on the television, I just hate it. It's not the film itself; it just reminds me of the way I felt at that time. I was sitting with my family watching the television and had a horrid feeling of dread for no particular reason. Then, all at once, my legs turned to jelly, my heart started racing and I felt like I couldn't breathe. The TV was suddenly too loud and the room felt like it was getting smaller. I remember going to the kitchen where I stayed for ages in floods of tears trying to deal with it on my own.

My friends and family knew that something serious was up because I wasn't eating. I felt too sick with the anxiety and was losing a lot of weight. I saw a lady about it, but I don't remember much because I think I have blocked it out. It is just a blur of anxiety and unhappiness to me. I don't remember the day I started to feel better. I guess I just started to be able to cope with it more. I still have anxiety but on a much more manageable level. As I've become older, I've discovered so many people suffer from anxiety on so many different levels and everyone's experience is unique but that there are many ways to deal with it. I will talk more about my experience and how I have learned to cope with these feelings later in the book.

The next chapter of my life was a really happy
one. In my last year of high school, I had loads
of friends and was studying hard for my GCSEs.
My favourite subjects were English and Drama.
I wasn't that confident, so performing in plays was
great because I could get into another character.

On weekends, I had a job at a shop called
Paddock Farm Shop in a nearby village. I know it
doesn't sound very exciting, but the owners were so
relaxed and I got to open and close the shop by myself
and I felt very responsible. Mum would drive me there
because it was in the middle of nowhere at about 8.30 a.m.
to open for 9 a.m. They had a massive, scary fridge at the
back about the size of a room, which had a huge metal
door. All the fruit and vegetables would be stacked up in
baskets and I had to take them out to stock the shelves.
Then I served customers all day. I was there on my own
and often it was quite quiet. We had a wind-up radio and I
regularly sat for a couple of hours without anyone else
coming in. Sometimes I did my homework or read books,
but I always remember texting boys and freaking out
because the phone signal was so bad. When there was no
one around, I would leg it to the main road and back again,
in case I could get a tiny bit of signal to see if they had
texted back. At 6 p.m., it was my job to put all the empty
baskets back in the fridge, but I was terrified of falling in
and the door shutting behind me. It was like something
out of a horror film, where they keep severed heads! All in
all, it was a fun Saturday job and I liked saving up to buy
myself treats. On the weekend evenings, I always had my

friends over for sleepovers and my parents say there was always an extra body at the end of my bed in the mornings.

In the run-up to my GCSEs, I had glandular fever and it was awful because I just felt so tired the whole time. Even when my friends called the house phone to speak to me, I was too tired to pick up and just lay in my bed or on the sofa feeling rubbish. As a result, I didn't do much revision for my exams. I wanted to go to my exams in my pyjamas but, obviously, I wasn't allowed! In the end, I did make it in and finished high school very happy with four A grades and six B grades. I celebrated a month later by dancing the night away with all my friends at the school prom.

Maddie and I went to a sixth form college in Norwich city centre called Notre Dame. Tasha, Kate and Emma were still at high school but we made a great group of friends, including Vanessa. I remember on my first day, we were all sitting on the floor in the reception area and I saw Vanessa. We made eye contact and she looked really friendly. I went up to her and said hi and we quickly became friends. I studied English, Classics and Psychology for A-Level. During the first year, I didn't have a very good time because I had another bout of anxiety and ended up missing quite a lot of my lessons.

By the time the second year came round, I was starting to feel quite uninspired by learning, but Kate who had been in the year below in high school came to Notre Dame and we were so happy to be together. I just gradually stopped feeling so anxious. We really got into music and started going to loads of gigs at UEA, where they have a big auditorium. We were really into indie music, like Larrikin Love and The Rifles. After I started earning pocket money at the farm shop, I liked being able to buy myself clothes and I got a job at Starbucks at the weekends.

One night Kate and I went to a house party, which was hosted by a guy we'd met at a Babyshambles concert the week before. Not realising that cool people only went to house parties at about 10 or 11 p.m., we turned up super-early at 8 p.m. and a cute guy wearing braces (holding up his trousers!) opened the door and he spent the whole night talking to us, so we didn't look like losers who had no friends. That guy's name was Jim. It turned out he had been in the year above me at my sixth form college but we had never met. He says now he remembers some of my friends but not me and that I didn't recognise him! We had loads of fun that evening and swapped numbers and agreed to be friends. I obviously didn't realise it back then, but that chance meeting with Jim would change everything.

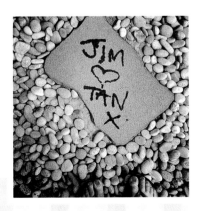

MY TOP 10
NOSTALGIC CHILDHOOD MEMORIES

1 | WHEN HEIDI AND MOLLY HAD PUPPIES

I was terrified of dogs when I was tiny. My grandparents on my dad's side were dog breeders and we used to see them a lot, too. I was always a bit scared of the hundreds of dogs at their house, so to help me get over being afraid, my parents got a King Charles Cavalier called Heidi. Later we got Molly and they both had puppies. Mum was like the midwife in our conservatory and I watched both sets of puppies being born. Heidi's waters actually broke on me when I was cuddling her! I remember one of Heidi's puppies was really tiny and we didn't think it would make it, but Dad wrapped some cotton around its belly button really tightly and it survived. We called it Cotton and it ended up being the fattest puppy in the litter!

2 | MAKING PLAY-DOH PEAS

When I was little, we used to spend hours playing with Play-Doh at our dining room table with all the children my Mum child-minded and it never lost its appeal. Mum always made her own version with flour, salt, oil and water and would then add food colouring and we had one or two different colours each week, which she would keep in Tupperware pots in the fridge to keep them soft. I recall making a lot of peas and carrots!

3 | THE MAGIC OF CHRISTMAS

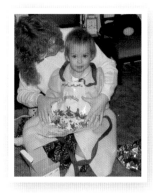

Christmas morning as a child was so magical. Before we went to bed, we put out a mince pie and brandy for Father Christmas and a carrot for the reindeers on the mantelpiece and then went upstairs and laid our stockings out on the ends of our beds. I vividly remember waking up in the middle of the night and seeing the stocking full of presents. That feeling of excitement is just one of the best! Even now I have to ask Jim or Mum to make sure they put my stocking out while I'm asleep, so if I wake up in the night I will be able to see it. One year, when I was about six, I wanted a really special toy bear I had seen and also this massive bar of Cadbury's Dairy Milk in Woolworths. To me it seemed about half a metre long, although it probably wasn't that enormous, but I just had to have it! I got both those things and I was so happy. I ended up naming the bear Curly Bear.

In the morning, Tasha and I would always take our stockings and open them in my parents' room. After that, we would go to the top of the stairs because the tree was at the bottom; we'd see loads of presents there and know Father Christmas had been. Mum and Dad would turn all the lights out apart from the ones on the tree, so it was like something from a Christmas film. Nanny and Granddad would drive over and we'd have bacon rolls and croissants for breakfast and open all our gifts. Later in the day we would go over to my nanny's and she would cook a traditional lunch with turkey and all the trimmings. I still think it is the best meal ever!

4 | SNOW DAYS

When we were off school because of the bad weather and snow, some of the children in the village would come round to our garden, where we would start massive projects like building a fort out of snow. Sometimes, we jumped over the fence at school and built a snowman in the field behind it. Afterwards we would cuddle up on the sofa and watch films or make pancakes. I still love it when it snows.

5 | GRANDDAD'S EPIC BEDTIME STORIES

If we stayed at my grandparents' house overnight or if they were at our house at bedtime, Granddad read to us and often he made up stories. They were always totally epic and he would include us as characters and places that we knew, which made it extra-special!

6 | WHEN KATE MOVED TO TASBURGH

When my friend Kate moved to Tasburgh, Emma and I decided she seemed like a lot of fun – a really nice girl that we wanted as our friend. We wrote her a letter saying, 'You're more than welcome to be our best friend now', and gave it to her at the bus bays in the school. She invited us to her house and told us her address but didn't say when to come round, so one day Emma and I just decided to set off from where we lived in Upper Tasburgh to her house in Lower Tasburgh. It was quite a walk and took us about half an hour. When we turned up, the house was gorgeous and had a huge back garden with a trampoline and no gate between the front and the back. We knocked on the door and no one answered, but we couldn't resist playing on the trampoline, so we went round the back and started playing on it. Suddenly all these cars pulled up on the driveway and all her family and extended family started getting out. It turned out that it was her dad's birthday and they had been out for lunch to celebrate. Her mum had no idea who we were and probably wondered what was going on! Kate explained and we were then invited in for birthday cake – I don't think they had much choice! We have been best friends ever since.

7 | DARTMOOR STEPPING STONES

While we didn't have any foreign holidays when we were growing up, sometimes we went to stay with my godparents, Veronica and Peter, who I was super-close to. They lived down in Devon and we travelled on the train together and stayed at their house. We spent our time on Teignmouth Beach and looking around the nearby villages, but my all-time favourite thing to do when we were there was to go to Dartmoor. We did lots of walking and hill climbing and sometimes went paddling at Spitchwick Common. My highlight, however, were the stepping-stones across the river near Badgers Holt. They are huge stones that form a bridge from one side of the river to the other and you have to be really careful that you don't fall in. It always felt like a real adventure.

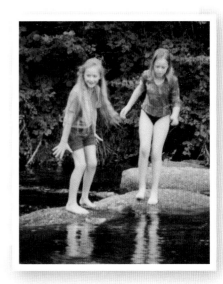

8 | THE AMAZING DRESSING-UP BOX

We often went to Banham Zoo when we were little, and at the weekends there would be a car boot sale in the car park. So while Mum took us to see the animals (apparently I was obsessed with the penguins!), Dad would wander around the sale and come back with loads of things for Tasha and I, like original Charleston hats, floppy felt hats from the 1970s and authentic vintage brooches. When we did our plays, everyone would use clothes from the special dressing-up box.

9 | BIKE RIDES TO NANNY AND GRANDDAD'S

Nothing was ever casual with me; I was always looking for a project of some sort. Every time we cycled to Nanny and Granddad's with our little group of friends, I would try to make us beat our previous timing. One day during the school holidays I had my friends to sleep over because I wanted to cycle there at 6 a.m. the next day. I was determined to do it and made Emma and Tasha stay on the floor in my room so I could wake them up with cold flannels! When we arrived at Nanny and Granddad's at 6.30a.m., they were a bit surprised to see us.

10 | SOUTHWOLD TIMES

We always used to spend a lot of time at Southwold, which is about forty minutes' drive from our house. The town has a beautiful, sandy beach and we spent a lot of time there growing up. Mum and Dad have a caravan there now and we try and stay there every summer.

NOTES

*List your top ten memorable moments
with your family...*

- -

- -

- -

- -

- -

- -

- -

- -

- -

- -

- -

- -

- -

- -

- -

♡

NOTES

List your favourite school memories...

♡

NOTES

List your top ten childhood heroes ...

♡

MY TOP 10
SONGS
THAT WOULD BE THE SOUNDTRACK TO MY LIFE GROWING UP

Like most people, music is a big part of my life. Writing this list of tracks was really hard because there is so much music that I listened to growing up, but I've tried to pick the top tunes that remind me of childhood and my teenage years.

1 | **RIGHT SAID FRED: 'DEEPLY DIPPY'**
This song reminds me so much of my dad when I was little. I wouldn't be surprised if he had sung it to me every day. He used to put on quite a performance, with all the different voices, high bits and crazy moves!

2 | **THE BEATLES**
It's impossible for me to pick out one of The Beatles' songs because we listened to their albums all the time at home. Both Mum and Dad were massive fans and Dad was always singing around the house. The tracks that stand out the most are 'All You Need Is Love', 'Help' and 'I Want To Hold Your Hand'.

3 | **THE BANGLES: 'ETERNAL FLAME'**
I knew the lyrics to this when I was so young and Mum thinks it is because she used to listen to it the whole time she was pregnant with me. We had it on an old-school tape and used to play it on repeat in the car.

4 | SPICE GIRLS: '2 BECOME 1'

I loved the Spice Girls and wanted to be Posh Spice. I remember watching their videos and trying to impersonate all of Posh's dance moves.

5 | RADIOHEAD: 'KARMA POLICE'

When I was a bit older, I had this on repeat in my bedroom constantly and would play it on my MP3 player on the bus with my friends. As a teenager you have a lot of crazy emotions and it was like this song had been written for my fourteen-year-old self.

6 | NIRVANA: 'SMELLS LIKE TEEN SPIRIT'

This was a house party song that I would always put on when we went to house parties when I was a teenager. I was crazy about Kurt Cobain.

7 | KELLY CLARKSON: 'BEHIND THESE HAZEL EYES'

This makes me think of working in the farm shop because it used to come on the radio a lot and I would carry my wind-up radio singing along at the top of my voice when no one was around. The shop was divided by an archway and on one occasion, I was in the back and I was belting it out, and when I got to the front, there was a queue of customers. So embarrassing!

8 | ELLIOTT SMITH: 'ANGELES'

After school most days, my friends and I talked to each other on MSN Messenger. When you went online you could see who was online and what music they were listening to. That was how I developed a lot of my music loves as a teenager, including this song.

9 | BLOC PARTY: 'BLUE LIGHT'

I love the entire *Silent Alarm* album but this track is my favourite. It reminds me of around the time I first met Jim and when we used to hang out together in the early days. Kate and I went to a Bloc Party gig at UEA and weirdly it was before I met Jim, but Kate remembers him being there.

10 | COLDPLAY: 'SPARKS'

This is my song with Jim and we used to listen to it all the time. He always used to write the lyrics 'I saw sparks' in cards he wrote for me. I have saved them all.

NOTES

List the top ten songs that would be the soundtrack to your life growing up...

♡

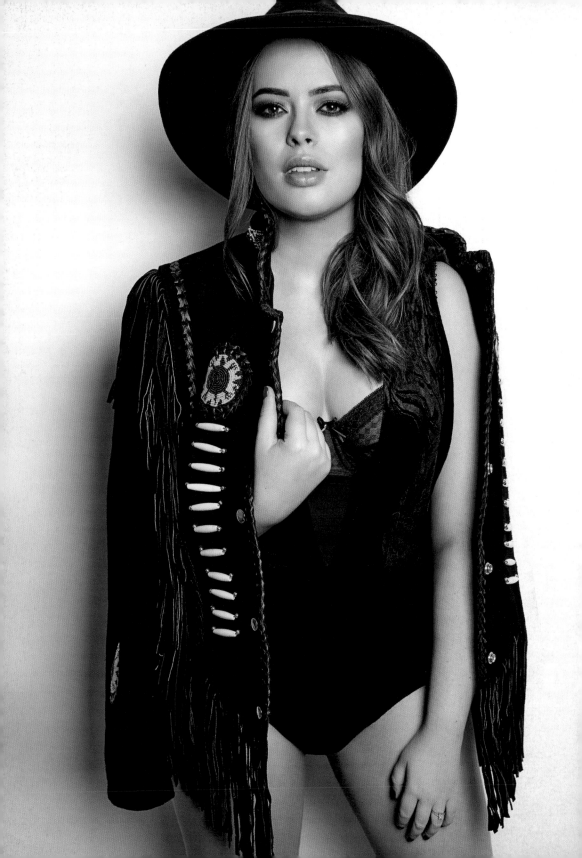

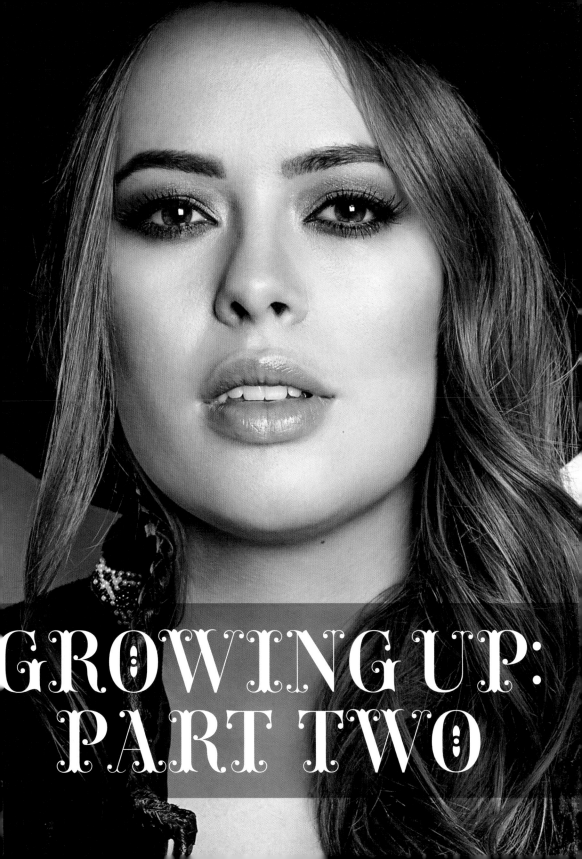

GROWING UP: PART TWO

Quite soon after meeting Jim, we became an item and fell in love. He was studying for a psychology degree at UEA and was living at home in Norwich and we spent a lot of time together at his house. From the first time I went to his family home and met his mum Judy, twin brother John and older sisters Sam and Nic, I loved being there. The house was always busy and everyone had their partners over all the time. Having always been the oldest one at my home, it was nice to be somewhere where I was the youngest.

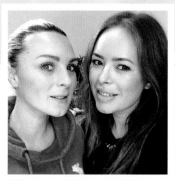

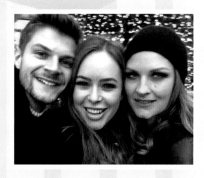

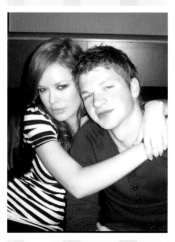

Jim's sisters Sam and Nic, who are about ten years older than him, are trained make-up artists. At the time Sam had just had her daughter Lily so I never saw her wearing make-up, but I looked at her work around the house and her make-up portfolio, which was incredible. Flicking through the pages and seeing all the different looks she had created, I was so impressed. Nic was working at MAC at the time in the city centre and her make-up was always flawless; she never looked anything but stunning.

On one of the first occasions that I stayed over, I realised that I hadn't brought any face wipes with me to take off my make-up. When I asked Jim if he could get one for me from one of his sisters, he told me to ask them myself. Slightly nervously, I went into Nic's room and along with some face wipes, she asked me if I wanted some make-up for the next day. I remember not being that bothered, thinking it might be a bit of concealer or something but she gave me a full face of amazing high-end make-up, including a MAC Mineralize Skinfinish, which was all glittery. She let me keep the compact and I still have it in my make-up collection now, though I should probably throw it out as it's so old!

Nic did my make-up for me for my sixth form prom and it was one of those 'wow' moments. I was completely transformed and felt really pretty for the first time ever! Apparently I always asked them loads of questions about how they achieved different looks and why certain products were better than others. I remember once we were going on a family trip to one of Jim's aunties for a barbecue and Nic was doing her make-up in the front of the car and I was sat in the back mesmerised by what she was doing. I knew then that I needed to learn to apply make-up like that for myself.

Originally I had planned to go to Leeds University to study for an English degree and had applied and got in but, by that point, I knew I wasn't going to go because beauty and make-up was the path I wanted to take. It was a big risk but I'm so glad that I took it. I started to assist Sam and Nic on jobs, like weddings at the weekends, and at other events, such as London Fashion Week shows and TV shoots. I found the whole experience of being on set so exciting, inspiring and creative. There was always cool music playing in the background and I was in awe watching Sam and the photographers at work. It felt like the type of environment that I would love to work in. Sam and Nic ran five-day intensive make-up courses and I went on one and learned so much. They also gave me loads of one-on-one lessons.

By then, Jim and I were inseparable and spent all our time at his house as it was closer to his university and the town centre, where we both worked. His mum Judy became like a second mum to me. In the centre of town, there is an independent department store called Jarrolds where Judy worked in women's fashion, Jim had a part-time job in the art department on the top floor and Nic was working at the MAC counter in the make-up department. They all said that it was a good place to work and that the staff were treated really well, so as soon as I left school I decided to get a job there. Obviously, I really wanted to work on one of the cool make-up counters like

MAC or Laura Mercier, but those jobs were pretty hard to come by. The first job that came up was on classic toiletries, where they sold brands like Roger & Gallet, Floris and Yardley. Judy and Nic advised me that if I worked there I would be right by the make-up and so I would be the first to know about any job openings. Also, that if I showed them I could work hard, then I would give myself the best chance of getting a job on one of counters. So I applied for the job and was offered it.

While I was working on classic toiletries, the first job that came up was on the MAC counter. I had my heart set on it and when I didn't get it, I was devastated. But after only three months on classic toiletries, a job came up at Laura Mercier. The brand is really creative, Laura Mercier is really hands-on and, unlike lots of other beauty brands, they really teach their staff about their products and how to apply them. Everyone who works there is called an artist, rather than just a salesperson, which was important to me as I was much more interested in the creative side than selling products. If you use great make-up techniques, that sells the product itself! When I was offered the job I was delighted and, very quickly, I felt like I was learning loads. They had these fantastic make-up artists, who freelanced for Laura Mercier and who came up from London to teach the staff about using their products. There was one girl in particular, called Katy, who really helped me a lot with things that I didn't feel very competent in. I always used to use all the customers to practise on. For a while I struggled with applying liquid eyeliner, so one Saturday I thought I would spend the

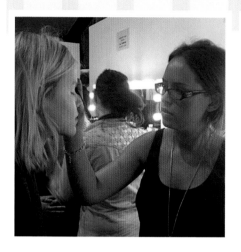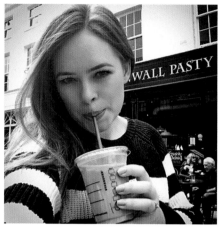

whole day asking if customers wanted to sit on my stool and have their make-up done so I could practise. That day I sold quite a lot of liquid eyeliners!

I ended up working on the Laura Mercier counter for two and a half years. While I hope I always did a good job with regards to the make-up, I always used to get into trouble for chatting too much! It was the same in every job. Mum reminded me the other day that when I was working at Starbucks, I was never particularly good at the job because I was quite slow at making coffee and I'm not that tidy, so I was never that good at cleaning up. However, I always enjoyed talking to the customers and some of them only wanted me to serve them. There were three Starbucks in Norwich and they always put me in the one that they thought would be the quietest!

I loved my time working at Laura Mercier and it felt like a real learning curve. I always worked at the weekends, but that meant I would get a couple of days in the week off and I would go and hang out at the university library with

Jim and just read books, or I sneaked into his lectures with him and his friends. I officially moved into Jim's house one day after he pointed out that it would make sense for me to have a few things there because I was there all the time.

Most days, Judy, Nic and I walked to Jarrolds together and if Jim and I were working, we always tried to get the same morning break and lunch break – we begged our respective managers – so we could see each other. Sometimes we'd pop out to get something to eat but most of the time we would sit in the café at Jarrolds and have beans on toast. They also have the best scones in the world and I always had one for my morning break. In fact, thinking about it, I must go back and have one when I'm next back in Norwich!

I discovered YouTube when I had been working at Laura Mercier for about a year and a half. Sam had started uploading tutorials to help her and Nic's clients, then people started requesting celebrity-inspired tutorials. So in some of the videos where Sam wanted to re-create the look of a younger celebrity, like Hilary Duff, Scarlett Johansson or Megan Fox, she would use me as her model. I felt really flattered by this and loved the whole process. Sometimes the viewers would leave comments, saying things like, 'Tanya needs her own YouTube channel!'

Sam suggested that I should start filming videos, just to practise different looks and build up my confidence. I filmed my first-ever video in her make-up studio, which was cool because it meant that I could use all her products. I filmed it on the webcam on Jim's MacBook. After Sam had given me a few basic instructions, and with a lot of help from Google, I edited it and uploaded it. I know it sounds naive, but I didn't care if people watched it or not, and while I always enjoyed reading the comments, it was over a year before I even noticed the viewer numbers below the screen. YouTube just wasn't such a big deal back then. For me, I just thought it was cool to have a video I had shot online and it was a fun and creative outlet. My new project then became to get a little video portfolio of my favourite looks online.

When I started to get a bit restless at Laura Mercier, I decided to work with a different skincare and make-up company because I thought they could teach me even more. I thought it would be good to have a new challenge but, eventually, it ended up being a bad decision. I have no idea how, but they found out about what I was doing on YouTube and said it was a conflict of interest, so I left.

At this point, my YouTube career wasn't earning enough money for me not to do something else, so I got a job at Topshop. I was only working part-time, which meant I had more time to work on my YouTube channel and to do some freelance make-up work on the side. As I had got more confident, Sam told me that she thought I was good enough to have my own clients, so whenever she couldn't do a wedding because she already had one booked, she would pass it over to me. They paid very well but I was always really nervous beforehand. For my first wedding booking, I went on my own and it was in the middle of nowhere and I ended up taking a taxi, which got lost.

I found it really daunting and for a long time I preferred assisting Sam. After the first wedding disaster, Kate used to drive and assist me. I just wanted the company and the weddings were always out in the countryside, so she would pick me up in her car and we'd go together. I also did make-up for the odd TV shoot. I worked on a sofa advert in Bury St Edmunds and Dad came to pick me up. Everyone always rallied round to help me and I'll always be so grateful for that. As well as being obsessed with make-up, I loved the business side of it and being my own boss, even if it was slightly terrifying that everything was happening so quickly!

I was really getting into my videos then and would film every day before work, and I loved reading the feedback. Sometimes I would receive some negative comments on some of my videos and it did upset me, but it doesn't bother me at all now. After two months of working at Topshop, the subscribers to my beauty channel had doubled and I started making a bit of money through the ads on my YouTube channel. I had also built up lots of freelance make-up work, which was often at the weekends, and that helped me to pay my rent.

I started thinking about ways I could do different things. On my videos people always asked me what jewellery I was wearing, so I thought I could try and set up my own little business. Dad made me my own e-commerce website and I wanted to find a jewellery company that would let me buy their jewellery at wholesale price and sell it on my site. I partnered up with a company called Tallulah Tu and they were awesome. The jewellery was really lovely costume-type pieces, like statement necklaces, stud earrings and rose gold bracelets. I didn't have much money, so initially I could only buy ten pairs of earrings in each style, and I sold them for the same price they were being sold on the Tallulah Tu website. I wore the jewellery on my videos; it really took off and it was really frantic packaging up lots of boxes and sending them off. In the end, I found it quite overwhelming because I had to buy so much stock and I couldn't keep on top of the postage and admin. I contacted them and they suggested giving me my own page on their website and I could help design the pieces, for a royalty fee. I told Sam and Nic about it and they suggested I talk to their manager, a guy called Dom Smales, about it. I ended up calling him and asking his advice and so that's how I ended up being managed by Dom's company, Gleam. In the end, my relationship with Tallulah Tu fizzled out but I loved it at the time!

After Jim finished uni, we decided to go travelling. We had spoken for ages about taking three months out to visit Thailand and Australia, so I quit my job at Topshop. I wasn't too worried about work. I knew I could pick-up with the weddings and freelance make-up work when I got back, and I had pre-recorded enough videos for two video tutorials a week while I was away. I worked really hard to get them done and Kate, who was studying at university at the time, said she would upload them for me – what a star!

We had some real adventures when we were travelling

together in Thailand, which I'll talk more about later in the book. We have some amazing memories too – we made some great friends there and partied a lot. From Thailand, we travelled to Australia, where we stayed in Sydney and lived with my cousin for six weeks.

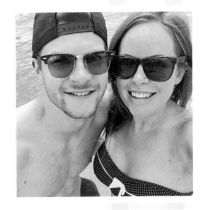

When we got back, Jim started making YouTube videos, too. He had a lot of free time on his hands while job-hunting. Originally he thought he'd like to be a primary school teacher but the job wasn't quite what he expected. He had some short-term contracts doing various things but, eventually, his YouTube work took off too, so we spent all our time making videos.

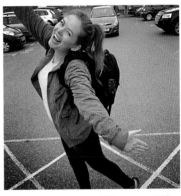

Before I went away, I promised my viewers that, after travelling, I would buy myself a new HD camera. All the videos until then had been terrible quality because they were done on my webcam. I got back on 6th January 2011 and told my viewers that by the 7th, there would be an HD tutorial online. It was a pretty big promise and the day I got back, I had dreadful jetlag, but I went straight out to John Lewis and picked up an HD camera. It looked so much better and it also revived my love of filming.

My YouTube channel was growing and I loved reading all the comments from viewers.I never really new where it was going to go; I just loved the connections that I formed with people. I loved filming, editing, making something look amazing and reading everyone's thoughts. I knew I had found a job that made me very happy.

MY TOP 10
EXPERIENCES THAT HAVE SHAPED WHO I HAVE BECOME

1 | **HAVING BIG PLANS**
Dad was always so entrepreneurial and did whatever he needed to do to provide for us. I think I've always been quite like him and am really business-minded. My granddad reminded me recently that when I was a teenager, I used to make long written plans about how I was going to build a business so I would be able to afford a flat overlooking Central Park in New York because I loved the TV shows *Friends* and *Sex in the City*. So you can see that I have always dreamed big!

2 | **CHOIR, PAPER ROUND AND MY SATURDAY JOBS**
Following on from what I've just said, I have always worked. I started off in the church choir when I was about ten. We would rehearse on Tuesday and Thursday evenings and then perform on Sunday at church and I was paid a pound every time I turned up. I remember one time when I was carrying the heavy cross up the aisle and it was so heavy that I almost knocked out half of the congregation! Sometimes I would ring the bells at church too.

When I was twelve, I got a job doing the paper round and it was really hard. The papers would always be delivered to the house and there were stacks of them. Every week it always felt there were more papers than the week before! The worst part was when they gave us piles of leaflets as well. I would have to get one of every single type of leaflet and put them in every paper. Then I would pack all my papers into this huge fluorescent bag and pop on my bike and deliver them and then come back to the house and fill my bag up and go out again, until every paper had been delivered. Then of course, I went on to work at the farm shop and at Starbucks.

3 | MY DANCE SHOWS
I would always be involved in all the shows the dance school I belonged to put on every year. We performed at one of the schools nearby that had a really big stage and we always got made-up with thick foundation and red lips. I loved the excitement of being backstage, and even though I used to get really nervous, I think being on stage has made me really confident and not worried about performing in front of lots of people. We also did competitions and when I was about eight, I danced at Sadler's Wells Theatre in London.

4 | MY LOVE OF READING
I have always loved reading. When I was tiny, Spot was my character of choice. I was very quick to learn to read and when I was about five, I loved this series of old-school LadyBird books called Puddle Lane. They came in five different sets, each one harder than the last. Mum

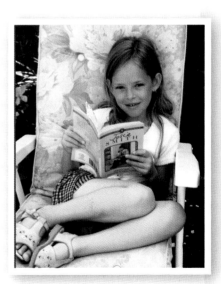

bought the first ones from a car boot sale but they were out of print, so we would always try and find more at charity shops and car boot sales and would be so thrilled when we did! At primary school, I would always read books at lunchtime and was put into the second year before my friends because I was such a bookworm. I read my first novel, *Pretty Polly*, by Dick King-Smith, when I was six. When I was slightly older, I sometimes read the books that Mum was studying for her degree, like *The Yellow Wallpaper* by Charlotte Perkins Gilmore, which was a bit weird but I enjoyed it. I have always read quite widely.

5 | ENJOYING THE SIMPLE THINGS

We had a simple childhood and didn't have lots of expensive toys or holidays and, even now, it's the little things that bring me the most pleasure. Using a pretty mug to drink my tea out of, being given a beautiful bunch of flowers or just spending time at home with my family bring me the most pleasure.

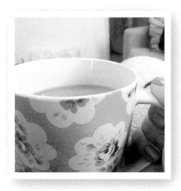

6 | HARRY POTTER

A huge part of my life growing up was about JK Rowling's Harry Potter series. I absolutely loved it. Tasha and I always made Dad take us to the midnight launches at Jarrolds so we could queue and be one of the first people to read the books the day they were released. I wouldn't leave the house and read each one in about two days. I was really obsessed with the whole series but particularly with Hermione. Sometimes, when I was younger, I used to be self-conscious about how bossy I was, but Hermione became such a role model for me and I think she made it OK for girls to take control. I must've read all the books about three times and watched the films ten times. I don't think my love of Harry Potter will ever disappear!

In May 2013, we went to the Warner Brothers Studio to see *The Making Of Harry Potter* with some other YouTube friends and it was the best day ever. I even got a picture of me flying on a broomstick!

7 | DRESSING UP

As I mentioned before, Dad used to buy us lots of vintage jewellery and outfits from car boot sales and I always loved dressing up with my friends. I think this has really contributed to my love of fashion and experimenting with clothes.

8 | THE INFLUENCE OF STRONG WOMEN

I feel like I've had some really strong women in my life. Firstly my mum. She's a lot stronger than she probably thinks she is, and she did an amazing job bringing us all up whilst working and learning to be a teacher. Jim's mum, Judy, is strong in different ways to my mum and has been an incredible positive influence on me. Lastly, I've been influenced by books I've read growing up. Due to what my mum was studying, I ended up reading quite a lot of feminist texts.

9 | EVERYONE BELIEVING IN ME

My dreams were never limited by anyone around me. All my family, friends and most of my schoolteachers have always made me believe that I can do whatever I want. Dad is so funny because I think he actually believes I could do anything I want to. If I said I wanted to be a singer, even though I have a terrible voice and definitely can't sing, Dad would say, 'Of course you can do it. We'll get you some singing lessons and you can be a star.' That is just what he is like. I'm a big dreamer and until now, if I've wanted to do something, I've always tried my best to make it happen.

10 | YOUTUBE

YouTube has really shaped my personality. It's given me so much confidence and encouraged me to be really open as a person. Before I started filming videos, I think I could be a bit awkward and shy in social situations but as I have done more and more videos, met more people and other opportunities have arisen because of my YouTube videos, I have become surer of myself.

NOTES

List the top ten things that have shaped who you have become...

♡

NOTES

List the people who have had a positive influence on your life and why...

- -

- -

- -

- -

- -

- -

- -

- -

- -

- -

- -

- -

- -

- -

- -

♡

NOTES

List your funniest or most embarrassing moments...

- -

- -

- -

- -

- -

- -

- -

- -

- -

- -

- -

- -

- -

- -

- -

♡

SKINCARE ESSENTIALS

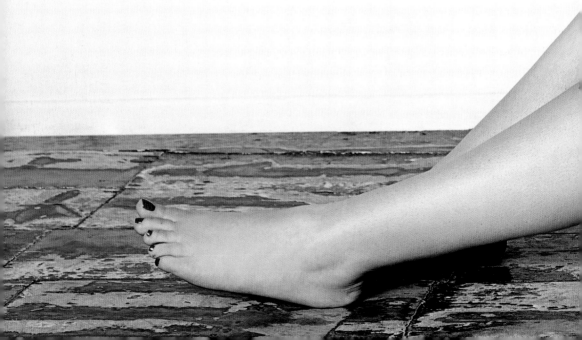

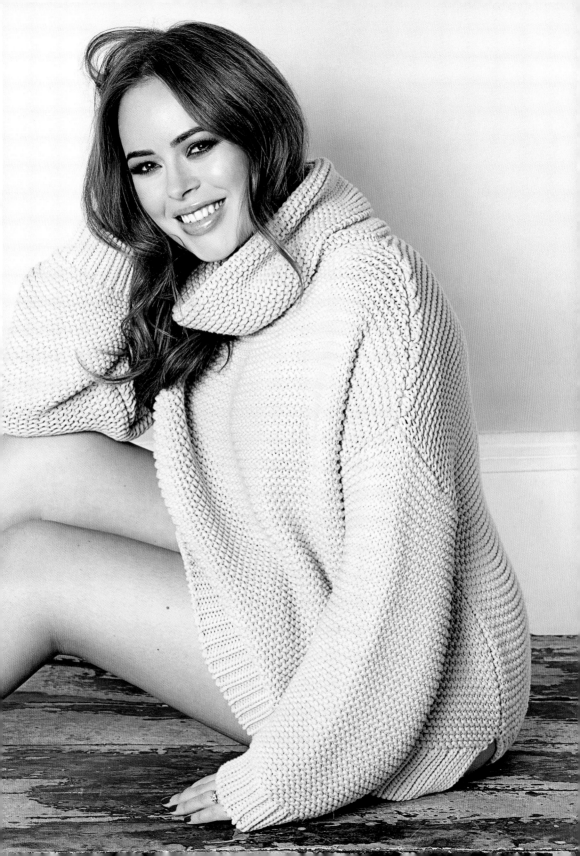

Beauty starts with smooth, healthy and glowing skin, so before talking about make-up, I thought I'd start by covering a few skincare basics. It's easy to look in magazines or on television and think everyone has perfect skin, but this really isn't the case at all – I promise! They often have expertly applied make-up on or the pictures have been lit in a certain way or retouched afterwards. Everyone has moments when their skin doesn't behave in the way they want. When I was younger, I was always so self-conscious if I had a little blemish or spot on my face and it would ruin my day. I'd love to be able to go back in time and tell my teenage self that I know it felt like the end of the world but no one ever notices! I don't tend to have crazy breakouts these days but I know when that happens it can really make you feel self-conscious. No one's skin is ever predictable and often hormones and other skin conditions are out of our hands. However, it is worth developing a good skincare regime because this can really help improve the condition of your skin.

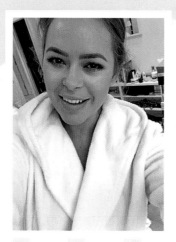

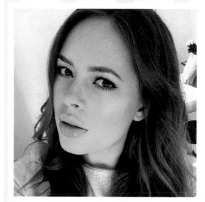

There are four basic skin types: oily, normal, dry and combination. They are all what they sound like: if your skin feels dehydrated and flaky, then you probably have dry skin; if your skin is often greasy and shiny, then you probably have oily skin; and if you don't have any issues with it, it is normal. Combination skin is where your skin type varies on different parts of your face or it changes and is a combination of dry or oily. I have combination to oily skin and get some shine around my T-zone, which is the area around my forehead, nose and mouth. It's called this because it is shaped like the letter 'T'.

When I was working on the Laura Mercier counter, I learned that in the UK, on average, we spend five minutes on our skincare and twenty-five minutes on our make-up, while in Japan they spend twenty-five minutes on their skincare and five minutes on their make-up, which is why all the people there have such amazing skin! Spending time on your skin really does pay off. My own routine isn't that complicated but it's taken me time to get to know what products work for me and you should do the same, so your skin always remains fresh-looking and glowing. When it comes to trying out new products or different brands, I would recommend that you decide on a set and use them for at least a month to see clear results. Also remember that your skin will change over time and you will need to update your regime on a regular basis in order to keep your complexion in tip-top condition.

CLEANSING

Cleansing is probably the most important, easiest and least expensive element when it comes to maintaining healthy skin. Cleansers remove bacteria, make-up, dirt and any oil that builds up on your skin during the day and will also help prepare your skin for any moisturiser or serums, so they can be easily absorbed.

There are loads of different types of cleansers to choose from and some contain more soap than others. I use a gentle cleansing balm that doesn't strip my skin of moisture and leaves it moisturised afterwards.

Apply your cleanser all over your face and use circular motions on the areas of congestion – the chin, nose and forehead – because this drains toxins. If you're using a balm or cream cleanser don't allow it to sink into the skin because it needs to remain on the surface to draw out impurities. Lots of people use an eye make-up remover first and if I'm wearing a lot of eye make-up I will too, but sometimes I'll feel too lazy to use one product to take my eye make-up off with and another to cleanse my skin. However, when taking your eye-make-up off with either cleanser or an eye make-up remover, it is always important to be gentle around your eyes and not to tug at the skin, because this area of your face is more sensitive and prone to damage.

Sometimes, if I have been wearing a lot of make-up, I love to double cleanse before going to bed. I put my cleanser on dry skin with a little bit of water, then take it off with a flannel and if my skin doesn't feel completely clean, I do the whole thing over again and my face feels amazing afterwards. It's really important to spend time while cleansing to remove all residue of make-up.

Finally, I should say never go to bed without taking off your make-up. Believe me, I often feel like I can't be bothered, especially when I've had a really long day! The thought of having to wet my face right before bed can be such a pain. So here's a tip in case you sometimes feel like that, too. As soon as you know you don't have anything else to do for the rest of the day, even as early as 6 p.m., take off your make-up, even if you're not going to bed until 10 p.m. Then it's like, yes! It's off! And you've done yourself a favour and don't have to worry about it at bedtime.

TONING

If I'm honest, I go through phases with toner and don't always use it, but if I find one I like it does make a real difference to my skin. I always keep a bottle of Clarins Gentle Exfoliator Brightening Toner in my bathroom cupboard for times when my skin feels really congested, as it always helps my skin feel clearer. It works by attracting moisture from the air and trapping it in the top layers of the skin. This product was recommended by Caroline Hirons – nothing better than a blogger recommendation! Aside from toner, I also like to use cleansing waters straight after cleanser because they remove any last traces of make-up and hydrate my skin.

EXFOLIATING

Exfoliators stimulate circulation in the skin and remove the dead skin cells, dirt and oil that get clogged deep in

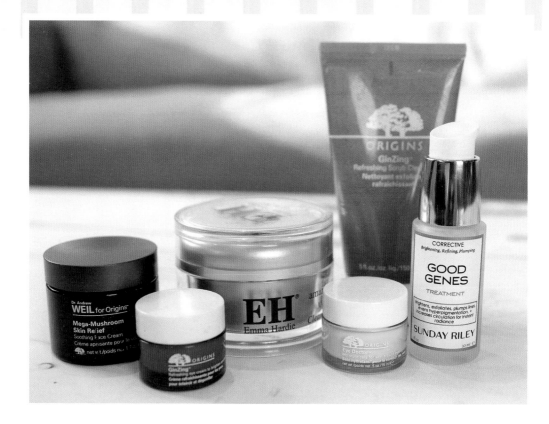

your pores. Some are harsher than others and if you have very oily skin, it can be tempting to vigorously exfoliate, but this can make the problem worse. All skin types can benefit from finer grains, more natural ingredients and spherical beads, rather than jagged grains. I use a gentle exfoliating cleanser in the morning which has jojoba beads in it which are spherical, and when you massage them into your skin, they don't scratch the surface but burst, leaving a light, moisturising oil on your skin. If you don't want a scrub you can get an exfoliating toner like the Clarins one I mentioned above. Exfoliating masks are another great alternative – Lush do some amazing ones!

SERUM

Serums are light and high-concentrated products that contain lots of anti-aging ingredients that are designed to get into the deeper layers of the skin. They can be worn under moisturiser or on their own and while they are more expensive than normal moisturisers, they do last for ages. When applying serum, only use a pea-sized amount because the skin will only absorb what it needs and after that, any excess product will be wasted. I started using serums a couple of years ago and I can really notice the difference in my skin.

MOISTURISER

Your skin type will play an important part in deciding what moisturiser you should choose because some are much thicker and creamier than others, but it is a myth that people with oily skin shouldn't use moisturiser.

Like most skincare products you don't have to break the bank because there are products available at every price point and some are really affordable. I love to give my face a mini-facial when moisturising. Warm the moisturiser between your hands to activate the ingredients, then use firm upward motions from the centre of the face towards the hairline. Don't forget your neck area!

EYE CREAM

This is good for keeping the delicate skin around your eyes hydrated and will help to combat fine lines. The skin around the eye is one tenth of the density of the skin on the face, so eye products are always much lighter than a moisturiser. I always say if you pinch the skin around your eye and then pinch the skin around your face, it feels as different as pinching the skin around your face and the skin on your forearm. You would never use your body lotion on your face, so you should never use your face cream on your eye area! Do pat the cream on or use soft, sweeping motions and give the cream time to absorb into the skin before applying make-up.

AND IF YOU SUFFER FROM ACNE OR BAD BREAKOUTS...

Let's face it: acne sucks! When I was younger I had the odd crazy breakout, and a few of my friends had more serious acne problems. They really hated it and thought that by using strong products they could literally scrub it off. But my recommendation for acne is, don't panic, and don't use tonnes of harsh acne products or pick your spots because those are the worst things you can do.

Instead, develop a proper skincare regime to prevent breakouts and maintain healthy skin. Always use oil-free cleanser with salicylic acid because this ingredient is anti-bacterial and helps to exfoliate away dead skin cells, which can clog your pores. If you find this too drying, use it two or three times a week alongside a calming and hydrating cleanser. You might find using toner worsens your breakouts or it might help; there is no one-size-fits-all formula, so sometimes it's a case of trial and error. Always use an oil-free moisturiser.

Topical over-the-counter products can help and your pharmacist will be able to advise you or, if you are really worried about your skin, visit your doctor because they will be able to offer you advice on the best treatments and getting help quickly can lessen the chances of being left with scars. Having acne can be tough and I know it might feel horrible, but with the right treatments, hopefully you'll be able to see big improvements over time.

A LITTLE NOTE ABOUT SPF...

Before I finish talking about skincare, I think it's important to also mention using SPF, because too much sun can be the skin's worst enemy. One thing we are all told time and time again is that while your skin might not show damage from the sun when we are young, it is really important to protect it when you are outside, otherwise it will catch up with you. I wear children's SPF factor 50 sun cream when I am on holiday and slather it all over my face, neck and chest to keep these areas protected. Sometimes it is easy to forget the top of your chest, but the skin here is also thin and therefore prone to sun damage. So always put on more than you think you need.

MY TOP 10
SKINCARE PRODUCTS

1 | **EMMA HARDIE MORINGA CLEANSING BALM**
I use this balm every night and it really gives my skin a deep cleanse without stripping it of moisture and feels really calming on my skin. The product contains grape and sweet almond seed oil, which are rich in fatty acids to help plump and soften the skin.

2 | **SIMPLE KIND TO SKIN CLEANSING FACIAL WIPES**
I don't think it's great to use face wipes all the time, but these are great when travelling and I always pop a packet in my bag when I'm on the go, for an easy and quick way to remove my make-up.

3 | **ORIGINS GINZING REFRESHING SCRUB CLEANSER**
This is a great wake-me-up cleanser for everyday use and I always use it when I'm in the shower first thing. It's really brightening because it is packed with radiance-boosting ginseng.

4 | **ORIGINS DR WEIL MEGA-MUSHROOM SKIN RELIEF SOOTHING FACE CREAM**
My face always feels super-hydrated after I have applied this rich face cream. It also really reduces redness, which I sometimes suffer from.

5 | **SUNDAY RILEY GOOD GENES TREATMENT**
This gives my skin an instant boost and makes it feel silky soft. It's super-charged with loads of vitamins and

active ingredients and I have noticed a visible change in my skin since I started using it.

6 | **BIODERMA CREOLINE H2O MAKE-UP REMOVER**
If I'm wearing loads of make-up, this is a great eye make-up remover because it is ultra-gentle, fragrance-free and manages to remove even the thickest mascara.

7 | **ORIGINS GINZING REFRESHING EYE CREAM**
I always apply this in the morning alongside my face moisturiser and it really illuminates the skin under my eyes so my eyes look really fresh, even if I'm tired or have had a late night.

8 | **ORIGINS EYE DOCTOR**
I always try to remember to apply eye cream at night and this one is really soothing and hydrating. It contains green tea extract, which fights off damage from free radicals, so will hopefully stop me going all wrinkly!

9 | **LUSH CATASTROPHE FRESH FACE MASK**
All my viewers will know that I am a big fan of all Lush products (especially at bath time!) and this face mask has blueberries, calamine and chamomile, and rose and almond oils to soothe and soften. It smells amazing!

10 | **KIEHL'S MIDNIGHT RECOVERY CONCENTRATE**
This replenishing skin elixir is for overnight use. I just apply a few drops to my skin and always wake up with supple, clearer skin when I've used it.

MY TOP 10
ESSENTIAL BEAUTY TIPS

1 | DRINK WATER

I know we're always told to drink eight glasses of water a day and it sounds quite boring, but drinking water is so important. If your skin is not getting a sufficient amount of water, it tends to become dry, tight, flaky and wrinkly. Drinking enough water will also give you increased energy, flush out toxins and make your skin look brighter and more radiant. So drink up!

2 | GET ENOUGH SLEEP

I always try to get my eight hours' sleep and if I've stayed at a friend's and haven't had a good sleep, I really miss it and crave sugary foods. If I don't have an event to go to or any plans in an evening, I always try to be in bed by 10 p.m. I think sleep is really important when it comes to feeling and looking good. Your skin and whole body go into repair mode when you're asleep and the skin renews itself. Lack of sleep can result in headaches, irritability, lack of energy and the inability to focus, and you will also find yourself more prone to breakouts. So get on your favourite PJs, snuggle down and have an early night! Use a soft pillowcase because this will be kinder to the skin on your face.

3 | EAT HEAPS OF FRUIT AND VEG

Try to incorporate lots of fresh food and vegetables into your diet. Some examples of foods that are good for your skin includes blueberries because they are packed with antioxidants and Vitamin C to help strengthen collagen formation; spinach, which is full of folic acid and vitamins; and sweet potatoes because these contain beta-carotene, which is great for your skin.

4 | GET TO KNOW YOUR SKIN

Everyone's skin is different. If you're unsure about what skin type you have or what might work for you, treat yourself to a facial. I've only ever had two facials in my lifetime but they were invaluable because I asked loads of questions and learned so much about my skin and the best products to use. A recommended facialist will give you all the recommendations you need to continue a good skincare regime at home.

5 | ALWAYS APPLY LIP BALM

Having flaky, chapped lips is not a good look, so do use your lip balm regularly to combat dry skin. I love sleeping with my Elizabeth Arden Eight Hour Cream slathered all over my lips, so when I wake up they feel really plump and hydrated.

6 | EXFOLIATE

Give yourself a full body exfoliation once a week. This is really important because it removes dead skin cells, improves circulation, helps with detoxification and is firming and toning. Basically it makes your skin look amazing! It is more effective if you apply the exfoliator or body scrub to dry skin, rather than when you are already in the shower. Massage the scrub all over your whole body from your toes to your shoulders and then get into the shower or bath and wash it away. Afterwards your skin will feel smooth and conditioned and you will feel like a completely new person!

7 | USE GRADUAL FAKE TAN

I go through real phases with fake tan; sometimes I prefer a paler skin look, while other times I love looking all sun-kissed and have a spray tan done by St Tropez. Having glowing skin can give you a real boost of confidence.

I always like my fake tan to look natural and I think the best way to fake tan at home is to use a gradual tan because it is less scary, with less room for error. Preparation is the key, so make sure you have exfoliated beforehand and pay closest attention to the dry areas of your body like your elbows. Work from your shoulders down and make sure you massage the product in really well. Always choose a specifically designed facial tanning product for your face. Afterwards, I wash my hands, then put a little bit just on the backs of my hands and rub them together, then rub my wrists together too. That way you don't have an obvious line between your wrists and hands. Give the tan time to dry and don't wear any tight clothes straight afterwards. It requires a few applications to achieve a good depth of colour and leaves your skin soft, moisturised and hopefully streak-free!

8 | MOISTURISE EVERY DAY

Make sure you moisturise your whole body every day, not just in the summer months when you're going to have more skin on show! Massage the moisturiser into your skin really thoroughly because this will improve your circulation and help you get rid of cellulite and it will also make you feel so much better about your body. And don't forget your feet – they need loads of TLC, too!

9 | BEAUTY ON THE GO

I travel a lot and whether it's a long car or train journey or a flight I'm on, I always try to go make-up-free so my skin can breathe. When packing, it's important to take your favourite products with you; just decant them into smaller plastic bottles. Flying in particular can really dry out your skin, so take your favourite hydrating face mask in your hand luggage. If you're meeting someone special at the other end of your journey, remove your face mask, then apply some tinted moisturiser, a slick of mascara and some lip gloss before you disembark and you'll look fresh-faced and gorgeous.

10 | GET THE GLOW

If you want more luminous skin from the inside out, work out three times a week. This will accelerate blood flow and bring oxygen and nutrients to the skin. Exercising will also help you detox, leaving your skin looking refreshed and regenerated. I know it can feel like a massive chore but it's worth it!

NOTES

List your skincare regime and the ways you might improve it...

- -

- -

- -

- -

- -

- -

- -

- -

- -

- -

- -

- -

- -

- -

- -

♡

NOTES

List your beauty icons and why they inspire you...

♡

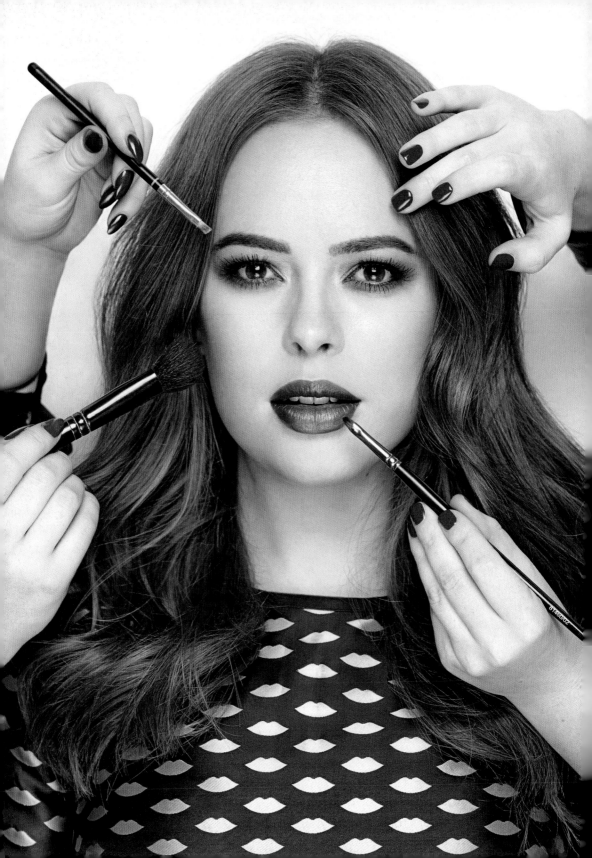

MAKE-UP ESSENTIALS

Make-up, to me, is all about creativity, expression and having fun. I love the fact that make-up can represent how you feel on any particular day and really help to complete a look. If I have a day when I want to feel really feminine and stylish, I try to re-create Audrey Hepburn's look and if I was going out and wanted to feel like a sexy bombshell, then I would go for a Marilyn Monroe look. I love the fact that I can wake up feeling and looking like one person and then leave the house looking like someone else!

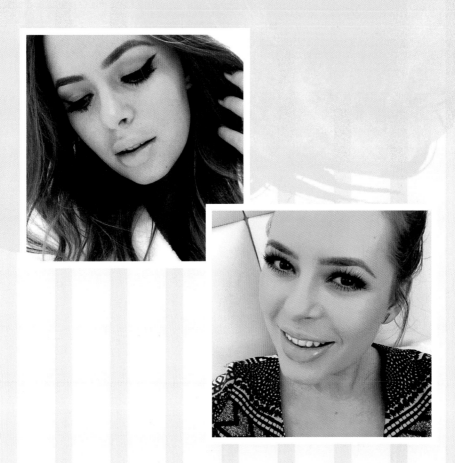

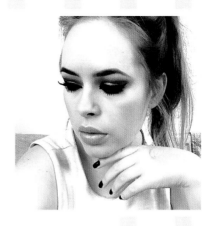

When I was growing up and as a teenager, I was always a real girly-girl and thought that make-up was fun, but I wasn't very serious about it. I remember having a Natural Collection Peppermint lip gloss and I used to keep it in my shirt pocket at school. When I was at my nanny and granddad's, we used to watch loads of old films, like *Seven Brides For Seven Brothers*, *Funny Face* and *Breakfast at Tiffany's*.

I always noticed how striking the actresses looked, and the polished look they all seemed to pull off perfectly is still one of my favourite make-up styles. Audrey Hepburn is my ultimate make-up icon because she looked so effortlessly chic and elegant all the time.

Since that time, my obsession with make-up has just continued to grow. I think that while experimenting and having fun with make-up is great, having just a small amount of basic make-up knowledge can have a huge impact on the way you look. I've decided to not cover different make-up looks because following them on my YouTube channel is easier (and I would still be writing this book in 2020!), but in this chapter I want to give you a few helpful tips and the absolute basics on applying a fresh face of gorgeous make-up.

TOOLS

Having the right kit makes all the difference when it comes to applying your make-up and, like any artist, a make-up artist wouldn't get anywhere without the correct tools!

BRUSHES

Even if you wear very simple make-up, it can look much better if you apply it with the right brushes. Good-quality brushes are not hard to find; almost every brand and many professional make-up artists have their own lines. While it might seem like a bit of an investment at first, not only will they give you a flawless finish but they will also help your products last longer as well as helping you save money in the long run. There are a huge range of styles, shapes and bristle types – you can choose from natural or synthetic ones – and I often change up my brushes and use different ones for different purposes. Here is a list of my top brushes that I couldn't live without.

Foundation brush

These come in so many different shapes and sizes. My favourite one – which is so good I think I'm going to use it for the rest of my life! – is the Bobbi Brown Face Blender. It's a fluffy brush that's not too dense and therefore applies foundation in the most natural way.

Blush brush

This is a round brush. It needs to be wide enough to cover the apple of your cheek and ultra-soft so it doesn't disturb

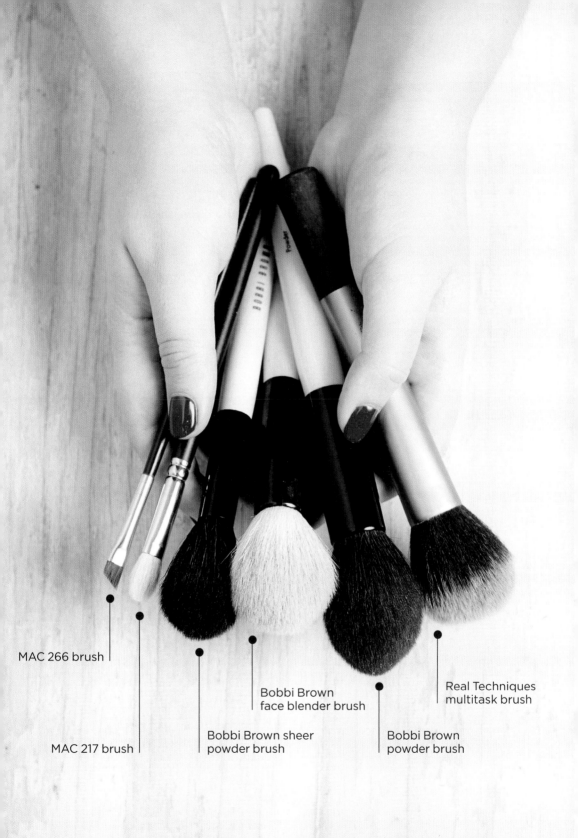

MAC 266 brush

MAC 217 brush

Bobbi Brown sheer
powder brush

Bobbi Brown
face blender brush

Bobbi Brown
powder brush

Real Techniques
multitask brush

your foundation or irritate your skin. My favourite at the moment is the Real Techniques Multitask Brush. I love using this brush because it has a nice round shape and is the perfect size for my cheeks. It's really important to get a brush that's the right size for your face. I have quite a big face, so when I'm doing make-up for my friends with smaller faces I have to use a smaller brush!

Bronzer brush
This is similar to a blush brush but it's good to have two so you don't mix up your colours.

Brow brush
I like to fill in my brows with powder or using a little gel pot and I don't use pencils, so for me this is a really important piece of my kit. This is a firm, angled brush that allows for optimal control when shading and defining.

Eyebrow spoolie
This is a bit like a mascara wand, minus the mascara! It ensures all your hairs lie in the right direction and will help to even out colour and soften any harsh edges after you have applied your brow powder or gel. Some eye pencils have built-in spoolies.

Concealer brush
Again, this is personal choice because many people like to use a narrow synthetic brush, where the ends are tapered to help you get to hard-to-reach spots. I like to use a

fluffier concealer brush, so it glides along my skin and blends the product in really well.

Eyeshadow brush

I like to use a soft, fluffy natural-hair brush that is good for blending eyeshadow into the crease of your eye and defining your lid with precision. My all-time favourite is the MAC 217 brush.

Eyelash curlers

I use my eyelash curlers all the time. Look for a basic metal version with ergonomic handles and rubber pads to help give your lashes a natural-looking curl before you apply mascara.

Powder brush

This is a big and soft, natural-hair brush for dusting powder onto the face. I really love the Bobbi Brown Powder Brush. It applies just the right amount of powder so I don't end up with too much.

Lip brush

This is a small round-tipped brush and will make precise lip colour application easy. It's great for applying strong colours, like statement red lips.

Tweezers

It's worth investing in a good pair of tweezers. I use these for helping me to apply my false eyelashes. As well as plucking out the odd stray hair, of course!

APPLYING YOUR MAKE-UP

How you apply your make-up totally depends on what look you want to achieve and I change up my make-up every day and go through phases of using different products, depending on whose look I am inspired by at the time. For me, anything can inspire a different make-up look, from a celebrity on the red carpet, to a cool music video, to someone that I see on the street with a striking image. Like most things, the more you practise the better you will become at applying your make-up, but here are some very basic facts and tips:

PRIMER

Before using foundation, it's good to use a primer. To be honest I don't always remember and have weeks where I forget that primer even exists, but at the moment I'm having a phase of loving it! It helps to minimise your pores, smoothes out fine lines and softens your skin, and it lays the base for foundation and will help it stay on your skin for longer. There are different sorts of primers for different skin types so choose one which is right for you.

★ Always apply primer after moisturising, otherwise your moisturiser will sit like a thin film on your face.

★ Don't coat your face with it – one small blob is plenty. Gently rub it all over the skin for even coverage.

★ Some primers are slightly tinted and can add a glow to your skin. Lilac shades brighten dull or sallow skin, while green or yellow tones neutralise redness.

★ Wait a few minutes before applying foundation.

FOUNDATION

The right foundation will make you look like you're not wearing any foundation at all. It shouldn't be a heavy mask and should just even out the skin tone and texture and make your skin look its best. There are so many different types of foundation on the market. Go to a department store and ask all the make-up counters to give you a few tiny samples or take along your own sample pot. Then try out a different one every day for a week. Take photos after applying in the morning, then at lunchtime and in the evening and see how it looks.

★ If you have dry or flaky skin, always exfoliate, cleanse and moisturise so the foundation doesn't accentuate your dryness. I used to have women come up to me at the Laura Mercier counter and say, 'I can't wear foundation, it looks so gross on my skin', but if you treat your skin correctly, then foundation works for everyone. I always used to have dryness around my nose, so I used cleansing oil, which helped to combat this. If your skin is particularly oily or prone to breakouts, choose an oil-free formula.

★ Always test the colour of foundation on your skin. If you are at a make-up counter, ask the staff if you can take their hand-held mirror to a window and look at the foundation in natural light because often the lights in beauty departments are spotlights and they don't give you an accurate representation of how natural the colour will look. The colour that blends into your skin colour is the winner!

★ Make sure you blend the foundation well at your jawline and down your neck. Work from the chin out towards the jawline and down onto the neck, making sure there is no visible line.

★ Never put a whole pump of foundation on your hand and stick your brush in it and put it on your face. Instead you need to apply it in fine layers. This will ensure you get a flawless look and you don't coat your face too heavily. If you think you haven't put enough on, let your foundation settle for a few minutes. Then blend or layer in more foundation in spots where it is needed. Ta-da! Job done.

CONCEALER

Sometimes foundation will cover all blemishes but I often find that the redness around my nose shows through my foundation, as well as the odd blemish and the dark circles under my eyes. For my face, I use something with slightly more coverage and I dab it on and then blend with a concealer brush. Under-eye concealers are creamier and more lightweight and should be one or two tones lighter than foundation so they brighten dark circles.

★ Dab concealer on rather than rubbing it in, because this will just rub it to a different part of your face. I find it really helpful to use a small, fluffy brush to blend my concealer in really well.

★ Yellow-toned colours are best for covering redness around the nose and on the face, while peach tones will cover any blue discolouration under the eye and bring warmth to the area. There is a full colour chart showing what colours cancel out other colours, so if you are unsure, look it up online or talk to a make-up artist.

★ Once I've corrected the colour under my eyes, I like to use a brightening concealer, which is often yellow-toned and helps to radiate light.

★ Like foundation, layer concealer so you avoid putting too much on. Wait a few minutes after applying the first layer and then look to see if more is needed.

POWDER

Powder creates a polished look and helps to keep make-up in place. I like to use a minimal amount of powder just to set my foundation and concealer for hours and keep my skin looking fresh.

★ Always use powder sparingly to avoid a 'white-out' look. I also like to use a sheer colourless translucent powder, like a blotting powder.

★ Not everyone needs powder. If you have particularly dry skin, only use powder to set your under-eye concealer.

★ Always be gentle because you don't want to push your foundation and concealer around your face.

CONTOURING AND HIGHLIGHTING

Contouring is where you can give your face more shape and make it look slimmer. It can help you bring out your cheekbones, slim your nose or subtly sculpt your face. Contouring can sound quite technical but the basic theory is that you want to use dark, matte shades on the areas you want to recede and absorb light. Apply it where you can see natural shadows on your face, like in the hollows of your cheekbones, your temples, around the hairline, or in the triangle under your chin, to slim the area. You can also do the sides of your nose to give a slimmer shape. Blend it carefully, so it just looks like a natural shadow. Highlighting can bring light back into your face, so use lighter shimmery tones on the areas you want to bring forward and reflect the light, like the top of your cheekbones, under your brow bone and in your cupid's bow. You can use cream highlighters, gels or powders. Again, the choice is extensive, so experiment and decide what you like best.

★ If you're going for a completely natural look, avoid any products with noticeable sparkles. But you can use the beautifully sparkly ones for that glowing Kim Kardashian look which I love.

★ Not all contouring and highlighting rules apply to everyone. It's important to keep your face shape in mind. If you are unsure, go to a make-up counter and ask them to show you how to perfect your highlighting and contouring method.

★ Practice makes perfect, so give yourself time to learn to do this.

★ Do always check your look in natural light to see that everything is well blended before leaving the house.

BRONZER AND BLUSH

Bronzers imitate the look you would get from being in the sun and are a way to add a healthy glow to the skin. I like to use bronzers for contouring and use a smaller, more angled brush but sometimes I like to use bronzer to give me an all-over glow, so I use a bigger brush to apply it. Blush will also create a healthy, pretty look and can make

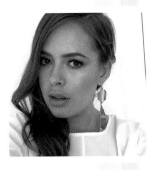

your skin look younger and your eyes brighter.

★ For a sun-kissed look, apply bronzer to the high points of your face – cheeks, nose and forehead, where the sun would naturally hit if you were on holiday.

★ When applying blusher, smile to find the apples of your cheeks and sweep upwards and outwards until no hard lines are left.

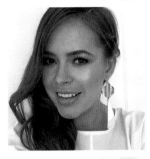

★ I always love to blend my blusher so that there are no harsh lines between where the blusher finishes and my skin begins. To achieve this, I use a powder brush or a foundation brush.

★ For the most natural blush look, match the colour to your cheeks when you are hot from exercise. But also, don't be scared to get creative with your colours. There are so many gorgeous blush colours out there and it's a case of seeing what suits you. A great thing to do is go to the make-up counters and experiment, as you might be surprised by the results. There's a colour by MAC called Frankly Scarlet which looks bright red in the pan but looks beautiful on if you use just a tiny amount.

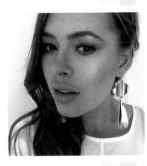

BROWS

Eyebrows are so important because they frame your eyes and will make a huge difference to your look. I am a huge fan of strong brows and I think all brows benefit from added definition.

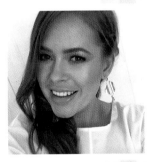

★ When it comes to getting the right eyebrow shape, I don't pluck my brows and my best piece of advice would be to go and get them threaded. It's an ancient technique in which someone twists cotton and uses it to pull out stray eyebrow hairs and it's less painful and quicker than plucking. You can get them done professionally quite cheaply. And even if you don't have the budget to get them threaded every six weeks, have them threaded once to get a good framework that you can then maintain yourself using tweezers.

★ It is also easy to tint your own brows, and brow tint kits are inexpensive. This will give you fuller-looking brows and they will be easier to colour in.

★ There are gels, powders and pencils to fill in your brow colour. My personal favourite is using powder applied with an angled brush for most precision.

★ When filling in brows, follow the direction of the hair in a flicking-up motion and don't use too much powder, otherwise you could end up with an unnatural look. I like to think of it as if I am drawing on little hairs.

★ Don't get carried away with tweezers – that's the worst thing you can do. But if you do, don't panic – you're going to get very good at filling in your eyebrows!

EYES: EYESHADOW, MASCARA AND EYELINER

Good eye make-up will accentuate the eyes and make your eye colour stand out. How you apply your eye make-up is entirely dependent on the look you are going for.

★ It's important to learn about the shape and positioning of your eyes so you can bring out the best in your features. For example, if your eyes are close-set you may want to use a lighter colour in your inner corners to make them appear further apart. My eyes are quite almond-shaped and I always like them to look as wide and open as possible, so I tend to blend my shadow into a rounded shape. If you're the opposite and prefer a less round look for your eyes, then wing your eyeshadow outwards. Once again, it's a case of experimenting and figuring out what works best for you!

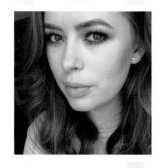

★ Before applying eyeshadow, I love applying a cream eyeshadow base because it creates a beautiful texture and a smooth canvas for my eye make-up.

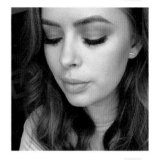

★ Always blend your eyeshadow well with a clean, fluffy brush across the area where your eyeshadow ends, to create a flawless finish.

★ I think classic black mascara is best for all occasions but pick your mascara according to the look you want. When applying mascara, don't pump the wand because this will push air into it and encourage it to dry out.

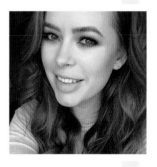

★ Work from the base to the tips of the lashes and roll the wand to avoid clumps. Always apply from underneath so you don't weigh down the lashes. Allow the mascara to dry before applying more coats if you want a more dramatic effect.

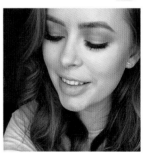

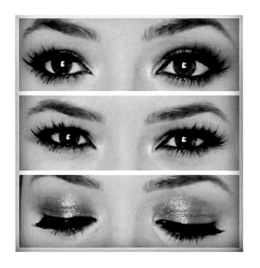

★ If you want a softer look, line your eyes with a powder eyeshadow using an angled brush. For a more dramatic look, use a gel or liquid liner to draw a line close to the lash line with a flick at the outer end. For an even more striking look, use a thicker line with a more accentuated flick at the end.

★ I love false eyelashes and have my own in my Tanya Burr Cosmetics range. I think they can really add to your look and open up the eyes and make them stand out. I'm a fan of more natural-looking false eyelashes. You can reuse them if you are very careful removing them.

LIPS

Applying lip colour is a simple but effective way to change your look. Again, there is a huge array of products, including lipsticks and glosses that are matte, sheer, shimmery and creamy. The right shades will complement your skin tone and work well with your natural lip colour.

★ Make sure your lips are well moisturised before applying lipstick. If your lips are dry, choose a tinted lip balm or gloss.

★ Use a lip scrub once a week to keep your lips smooth and kissable. You don't need to buy a special one: mix some honey with sugar or salt and gently rub onto your

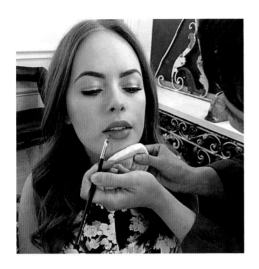
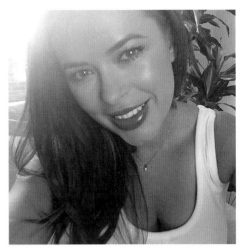

lips with your finger, remove it with warm water and finish with a slick of lip balm. Easy!

★ Personally, I'm not a big fan of lip liner but if you want to use it to define the shape of your face, pick a colour that matches the shade of the lipstick. If it doesn't match exactly, line your lips, then fill them in with the liner and put the lipstick on top, so you don't risk a noticeable line.

★ If you have a lipstick colour that you love but you think it's too strong, which is something that happens to me quite a lot, dab it onto your lips, then rub it in with your finger for a more natural effect.

★ Lip gloss is a great way to add natural colour to your make-up look, when lipstick feels too strong. I wear my Tanya Burr Cosmetics lip gloss in Chic almost every day.

MY TOP 10
MUST-HAVES FOR
YOUR MAKE-UP BAG

1 | **SHU UEMURA EYELASH CURLERS**
I use these all the time before applying mascara or false lashes because they give my lashes a really good curl. I like to put my lashes in, squeeze down and pump three times.

2 | **BRUSHES**
I have a range of brushes in different shapes and sizes. My favourite brands are Real Techniques, MAC and Bobbi Brown. Always make sure you clean your brushes regularly with warm water and a mild soap or shampoo.

3 | **URBAN DECAY 24/7 GLIDE-ON EYE PENCIL**
These pencils are soft and creamy and last all day. I hate it when make-up ends up halfway down my face and these never smudge. Roach is a flattering warm-brown colour.

4 | **HOURGLASS ILLUSION TINTED MOISTURISER OIL-FREE AND NARS SHEER GLOW FOUNDATION**
I've put these two products together because I mix them for the perfect flawless finish.

5 | **MAC PREP + PRIME HIGHLIGHTER PEN**
This pen-style highlighter has a light consistency but gives me great coverage and that Kim Kardashian glow under the eyes. It can be used over make-up for highlighting or under make-up to brighten and prime.

6 | TANYA BURR COSMETICS INDIVIDUAL LASHES

I'm never without my false lashes if I'm going out in the evening. They really open up my eyes and are great for taking selfies with my friends as they make my eyes look amazing in photos. I love my individual lashes because they look so natural. They come with glue in the pack, so all I need is my tweezers to apply them. Lay the lash on top of your natural lashes – the key is not to fiddle with it else it will end up on your finger!

7 | LANCÔME GRANDIOSE MASCARA

This mascara gives a real false-lash effect. The shape of the wand helps me fan my lashes out.

8 | BOBBI BROWN BRIGHTENING FINISHING POWDER

For daytime, this powder sets my make-up in place but instantly illuminates my skin and gives it a healthy finish.

9 | MAC MYSTERY EYESHADOW

I use this on my eyebrows and I really like the colour. I've got quite a bit of experience using MAC eyeshadows, as they were some of the first I purchased and I think they are the best. The pigment is amazing, they blend beautifully and the colour range is like no other.

10 | ELIZABETH ARDEN EIGHT-HOUR CREAM

This is the best lip balm and I have been using it forever. You can also use it to highlight your brow bone, cheekbones and even your legs. That's what I call multi-tasking!

NOTES

*List the top ten make-up looks you
are inspired by at the moment...*

♡

NOTES

List the top ten items in your make-up bag...

$\heartsuit$

MY TOP 10
BARGAIN BEAUTY BUYS

1 | **RIMMEL WAKE-ME-UP FOUNDATION**
This is really light and comfortable on my skin but gives great coverage at the same time.

2 | **COLLECTION LASTING PERFECTION CONCEALER**
This concealer covers even the worst blemishes brilliantly and lasts for a really long time on the skin. It says it lasts for sixteen hours and I don't think I've ever worn my make-up for that long, but I can believe it!

3 | **RIMMEL STAY-MATTE POWDER**
This product minimises the appearance of pores and provides natural-looking coverage. It's great to pop into your bag when you're out and about.

4 | **MAYBELLINE BABY LIPS TINTED LIP BALM**
These tinted lip balms are really hydrating, have a lovely sheer colour and smell amazing! They are not sticky at all and they stay on for ages.

5 | **MAYBELLINE FALSIES MASCARA**
This is one of my most-used mascaras because it really makes my lashes stand out and gives a false-lash effect.

6 | REVLON COLORBURST LIP BUTTER

This lipstick has super-charged hydration, so unlike some lipsticks that can be quite drying, it always makes my lips feel silky smooth. My favourite colour in this range is Pink Truffle.

7 | TANYA BURR COSMETICS NAIL POLISHES

These give a really professional, long-lasting finish and are chip resistant. When I created the line I wanted a range of colours to complement different outfits and looks. My favourite one at the moment is Riding Hood.

8 | BOURJOIS DELICE DE POUDRE

This bronzer has an ultra-soft texture and it's really easy to blend. It gives a really high-end, illuminating finish.

9 | L'OREAL SUPER LINER

I use this all the time to line my eyes. Some eye-liners can feel quite watery but this one gives a really opaque black finish.

10 | TANYA BURR COSMETICS LIP GLOSSES

I wear my lip glosses all the time and they are really hydrating. My favourite at the moment is Chic – it is the most gorgeous, neutral colour.

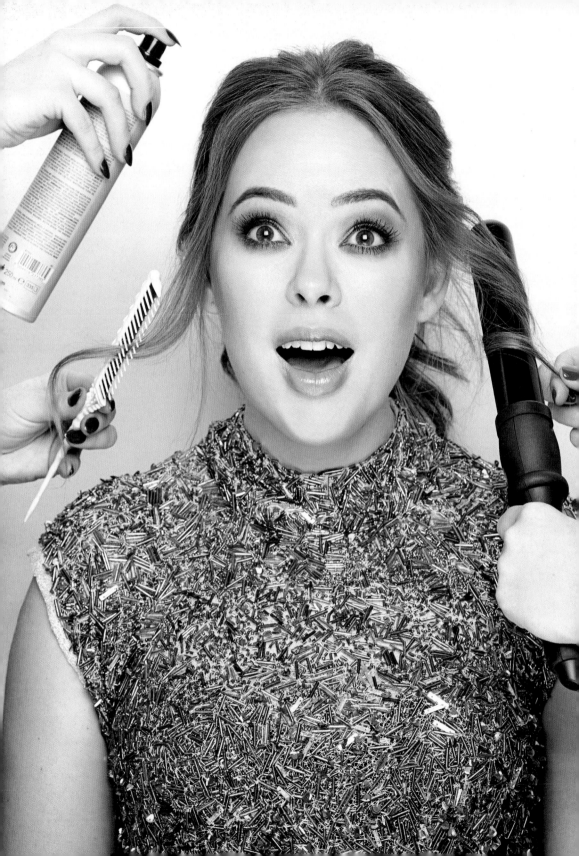

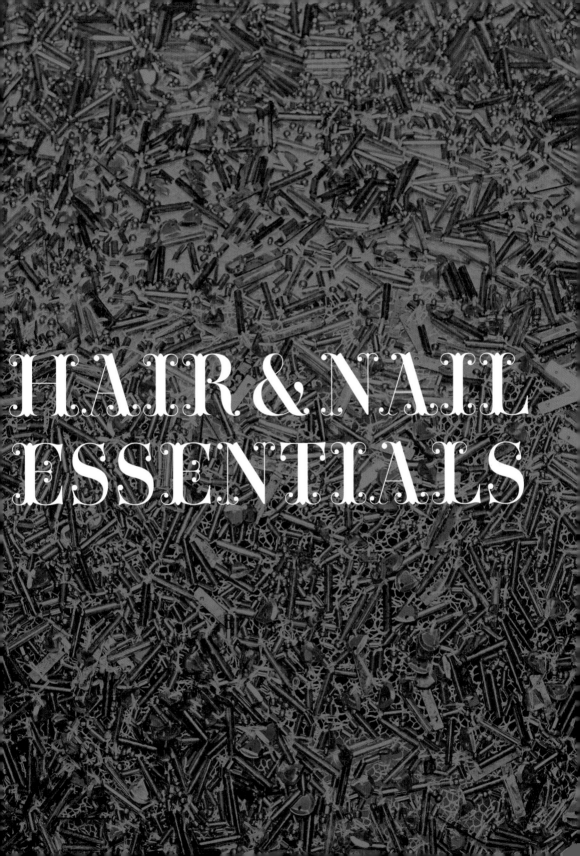

HAIR & NAIL ESSENTIALS

HAIR

Having great hair is all part of looking good. While my focus has always been on make-up, like any girl, I love to style my hair and have done since I was really small. Growing up, I always played hairdressers with Mum and Tasha. We had a box with all our hair accessories and we would be at it for hours. I even used to do my godfather Peter's hair and as soon as I walked away, my poor godmother Veronica would quickly try and put it back to normal again!

I've not always had long hair. Mum told me recently that when I was small I used to suck my thumb and twiddle my hair, which broke it all off. On one side of my head I had this bald patch, while the other side had hair, so Mum took me round to see her neighbour who was a hairdresser and she went over my hair with the hair clippers to cut it really short! Thankfully, this worked and I stopped sucking my thumb soon afterwards and it grew back!

Over the past few years my basic longer-length hairstyle has stayed the same and I have never wanted to play around with my colour, but I love having different styles. My hairstyle hero is Olivia Palermo because her hair always looks so polished and glossy.

As with fashion, I find myself inspired to create different hairstyles from a range of places. If I'm looking for new ideas, I love looking at pictures of people on the red carpet on Instagram and Pinterest and also just people on the street. So, for example, if I feel like I want to braid my hair,

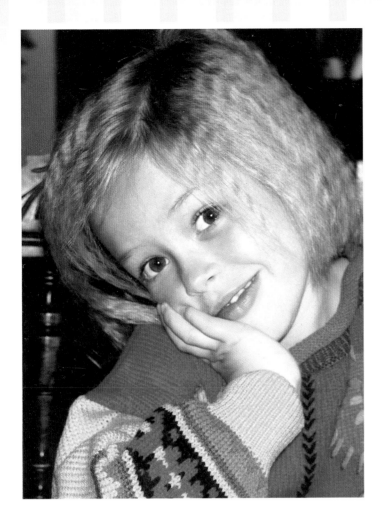

I type in 'braided hair' into Instagram and there will
always be hundreds of gorgeous styles for me to admire.

Sometimes I style my hair myself and on other
occasions my stylist Samantha Cusick does it for me.
I'm definitely not a hair expert but I love experimenting
with cool hairstyles. On the following pages are some
basic hints and tips that I have learnt, along with
some of my favourite looks. Enjoy!

BASIC HAIR CARE

A big part of great everyday hair, much like skin, is discovering what type of hair you have and what products work best for you. Most hair can be divided into roughly three categories: fine, medium and coarse. Understanding your hair texture and type, along with your face shape, can really help you figure out the best cut for you. As always, it's great to get the advice of a professional, so if you're thinking about having a new haircut, gather lots of photos or pictures of looks from celebrities or people that inspire you and take them with you to your hairdresser's. It's also worth considering your lifestyle: you may love a certain image but if you always roll out of bed at the last-minute then a cut that needs lots of styling probably won't be the right choice for you.

When you're at the hairdresser's, always be confident and say very clearly exactly what you want because if you don't, I find that some hairdressers will do what they want instead! I found Samantha by chance, but discovering the right person for you is always a process of trial and error. If you find a hairdresser that you love, stick with them, as they will get to know you and understand what you want from your hairstyle.

Also, I think it is important to spend money on getting your hair done properly at a salon. Sometimes when we were younger, my friends and I used to cut each other's hair and it was, without exception, always a complete disaster! I remember one time when I tried to dye my friend Emma's hair peroxide blonde and it went a rainbow of colours, including green and orange. Her poor mum had to take her to a proper salon where they were forced to dye it dark brown to correct it. It might seem extravagant, but I think that hair is one of the first things people notice when they look at you and it completely affects your overall look. Someone once said to me, 'Hair is like clothes, except you wear your hairstyle all the time', and that has always stuck with me.

When buying hair products, think about what you are trying to achieve, so it might be adding moisture, creating volume and thickness, smoothing and reducing frizz, protecting hair colour or enhancing curls or waves. Most brands will have basic shampoos and conditioners for every eventuality. The same applies to styling products: do you want to create texture and definition? Do you want high shine? Are you hoping for your hair to hold for longer, even when it is humid? Every big hair brand will have something for you.

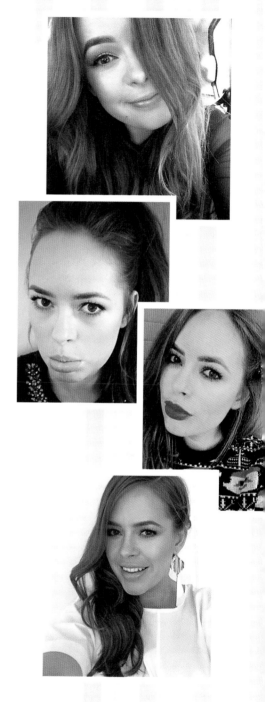

STYLING AND MY FAVOURITE LOOKS

There are hundreds of ways you can style your hair and I could fill a whole book with my favourite hair fashions, but here is just a selection of some of my favourite everyday styles and how to achieve them:

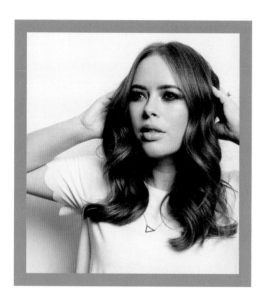

LOOSE, NATURAL WAVES

I love natural-looking hair with soft movement and I find this look is perfect for wearing every day as an alternative to normal, straight hair. To achieve this look I would use a curling wand with the same width all the way down (approximately one inch) on a medium heat setting. Then take fairly large sections of hair and wrap them around the curling wand, starting three-quarters of the way up so as not to get too much root volume. Hold for about five to ten seconds depending on hair type. Try to curl sections away from the face to create width. Repeat until all hair is curled. It doesn't matter if the sections of hair are different sizes or you do wrap it in different directions because this will help give your style a more everyday look. Run your hands through the hair to break up the waves and give that loose, natural feel. Finally, give your waves hold with a spritz of hairspray.

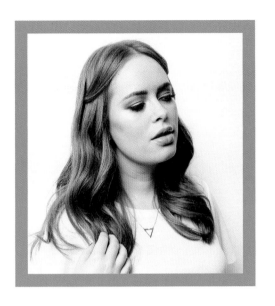

EASY AND CUTE PINNED-BACK HAIR

I love wearing my hair down but sometimes it gets in my face, so I like this look because it is easy. I love to curl my hair and you can do it like the waves opposite or on natural hair. I run a Tangle Teezer through the curls to make them look really bouncy and use hairspray to keep the body in my hair. Then take a section of hair from the side, near the front of your hairline, and using a butterfly clip or bobby pins secure it back and into place. You can also twist or braid these sections of hair back as a variation on this look. Repeat on both sides. I like to pull the strands of twisted hair out slightly, so they are not too tight into the head.

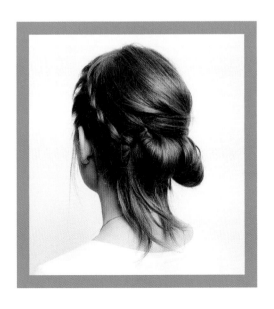

BRAIDED UP-DO

I really love this look because I rarely wear my hair up, so it makes a change and is a bit more special than what I do every day. I start by parting my hair in the centre and from the crown down to just behind the ears. Starting from the top hairline, French braid (see page 107) these sections to behind the ear, passing the strands over one another rather than under to create a braid that is not flat to the head, and secure with a bobble. Next, slightly backcomb the back section of hair just under the crown to create a bit of volume and then secure into a low ponytail. Pin the braided hair around the base of the ponytail to conceal that bobble and the rest of the braided hair. Then take the ponytail and roll it upwards, leaving the ends loose, and pin into place. Use a tail comb to tease out any bits that look too tight to the head, and hold in place with a global spritz of hairspray.

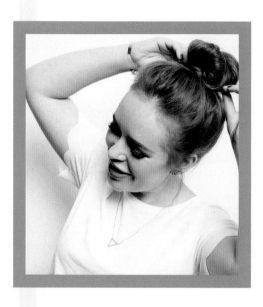

HIGH BUN

This style can be great for special occasions or everyday! You can make it as messy or neat as you like, depending on the occasion. I start by putting my hair in a high ponytail on the top of my head. Then grab the hair and wrap it around the base and keep wrapping until you have used all your hair. Pin your hair all the way around the bun to secure it. Sometimes I add some extra glamour with a hair accessory around the bun, like a string of pearls. I finish with a spritz of hairspray.

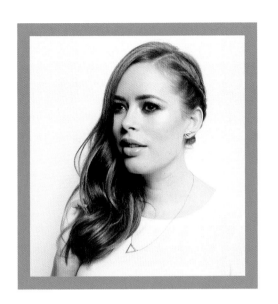

SIDE FRENCH BRAID

This side-swept plait is one of my favourite styles because it is really elegant. I wore my hair like this to the premiere of *Hunger Games: The Mockingjay (Part 1)* at the end of last year. To start, give yourself a deep side parting and section the rest of your hair off. To start a French plait, section this portion of hair into three even strands and start a normal plait. Once you have this small foundation plait, begin adding more hair to each section to form a French braid. With this look you want to pass the pieces under each other so the braid sits tighter to the scalp. Continue the braid right round to the nape of your neck, remembering to keep it close to your head. Secure the end of the braid with a band and then use a pin to attach this to your head and give it a blast of hairspray to hold it in place. On the other side of your hair, you can do whatever you want, but I like to wear my hair down and in loose waves.

MY TOP 10
HAIR RULES

1 | DON'T OVERWASH YOUR HAIR

I used to wash my hair every day but now I only wash it every three days and not only does this save me time, but my hair feels healthier. The less you wash and touch your hair, the less it breaks, and washing it all the time strips it of natural oils. The best way to cut down on hair washing is to cut down gradually. The first couple of times you do it, your hair might feel gross but slowly you will get used to it. Maybe on the second day curl your hair and add some dry shampoo, then after about a month you will be able to leave it an extra day before washing. On the days you do wash your hair, two shampoos before conditioning will help the hair feel cleaner in between washes.

2 | INVEST IN DRY SHAMPOO

These clever hair revivers deliver that fresh feeling without a drop of water and will help to reduce the oil build-up on your hair and give it amazing texture. Before spraying, shake the can well to distribute the powder and hold it at least six inches from your head. Lift up your hair in sections and spray the dry shampoo at the roots, and let it sit for a few minutes before styling. You can leave it in, instead of brushing it out, to give extra volume.

3 | DON'T USE TOO MUCH PRODUCT

The more products that you apply to your hair, the more you risk weighing your hair down and causing product build-up. Every couple of weeks, I shampoo my hair twice to wash all traces of product out.

4 | USE A HOME-MADE HAIR MASK

Do a hair mask once a week to keep your hair in its best condition. There's no need to buy an expensive one. Items that you might have in your cupboard that are great for hair include eggs, avocado, coconut oil and honey. Leave your mask on for fifteen minutes while you're in the bath, as the steam will help the mask to penetrate and repair the hair, and then thoroughly rinse the mask out before shampooing.

5 | SHAMPOO THE SCALP NOT THE ENDS

Use shampoo on the scalp only – not the ends of your hair. The shampoo will rinse down in the shower and cleanse the ends. This is especially important on longer hair that can get quite tangled.

6 | MASSAGE WHEN WASHING

Give your head an invigorating massage as you shampoo because this is a good way to encourage blood circulation and helps detoxify the scalp.

7 | RINSE WITH COLD WATER

After washing your hair, give it a blast of cold water. This adds shine because your hair cuticles reflect more light, making hair appear shinier and healthier.

8 | COMB WET HAIR RATHER THAN BRUSHING

When your hair is wet it is weaker and more fragile and susceptible to breakage. Start by gently pressing the water out of your hair with a towel and then use a wide-tooth comb or a Tangle Teezer and work in sections, starting at the bottom of the hair and working up to the roots.

9 | SLEEP WITH YOUR HAIR IN A BRAID

If you have long hair, sleep with it in a braid to avoid getting knotty hair and keep it loose for comfort.

10 | GET REGULAR TRIMS

Even if you're on a budget and growing your hair, get it trimmed every six to eight weeks to remove any split ends or damage. This will make your hair easier to style and manage and it will look so much better too.

NOTES

*List the hairstyles that you feel excited
by and want to try…*

♡

MY TOP 10
HAIR STYLING TIPS

1 | BLOW-DRY YOUR HAIR UPSIDE DOWN

Hang your hair upside down while you blow-dry because this encourages volume and creates a smooth, all-over fullness. Finish with a blast of cold air to seal the cuticles, boost shine and reduce frizz.

2 | USE PROTECTIVE TREATMENTS

These will provide the best protection for your hair while you style it. There are lots of different sprays and creams; some are especially designed to give you straight, shiny hair or curls, while others are created for more gentle styling, so select the best product for your needs. I also like to squirt a root-lift spray onto my roots before drying to give my hair a bit of extra volume.

3 | BRUSH FROM THE BOTTOM IN SECTIONS

Brushing thick hair from the roots can cause damage. Always brush from the bottom in sections and work upwards. My sister has really thick hair, so my dad always had to do this for her when we were little.

4 | DON'T GET STUCK IN A STYLE RUT

If you always seem to have the same hairstyle, head to Pinterest or YouTube to get inspiration for new ideas. If you're having a new style cut, take pictures or photos of the look you are after with you to show your hair stylist.

5 | USE MOUSSE

If your hair is too clean and slippery and difficult to style, use a small amount of mousse rubbed through the ends to give your hair some grip. You can even apply mousse to dry hair and blowdry it in to prep the hair for waves or an up-do.

6 | DON'T BE AFRAID OF HAIR EXTENSIONS

If your hair isn't particularly thick, don't be afraid of using hair extensions. There are loads of different types available and my favourite ones are Swift Hair extensions by B*long. They fit around your hair using a translucent wire, so there is no glue or clips and they don't damage your hair in any way. They are very easy to use and look completely natural.

7 | TAKE A HEAT BREAK

Rather than style your hair using heat, there are a variety of heat-less hairstyles you can try. If you want loose waves, wash your hair and when it is almost dry twist your hair into a swirly bun and secure it with a small butterfly clip at the top of your head at night. Sleep with it on and when you wake up in the morning and take it out you will have soft, natural-looking hair and lots of volume. The other way of getting slightly tighter curls is to do two braids on either side of your hair before bed again, when it is slightly damp. Continue to braid as close to the ends of your hair as possible, so the curls go right down to the end.

8 | DON'T APPLY TOO MUCH PRODUCT

If you're putting a serum, oils or leave-in conditioner into your hair, use less than you think you need. Put some product into the palm of your hand first and rub your hands together before running them through your hair, so that it is evenly distributed.

9 | USE YOUR STRAIGHTENERS FOR DIFFERENT STYLES

There is a heat styling tool for every look you could dream of, but if you don't have the budget to buy lots of different tools or you have limited storage space, you can create lots of different looks with your straighteners, including waves and many different styles of curls.

10 | NEVER USE STRAIGHTENERS ON WET OR DAMP HAIR

Have you ever put your straighteners on wet hair, only to hear a sizzling sound and see a cloud of steam? Straighteners get very hot and this amount of heat can cause the water inside the hair shaft to actually boil if you put them against wet hair, which in turn causes serious breakage and damage in that spot. Yikes! So always thoroughly dry your hair before using heat-styling tools. This includes when you use heat protection sprays – if you apply a heat protection spray to dry hair don't forget to blowdry it in!

NOTES

List your top ten favourite nail varnishes...

NAILS

Having beautiful nails feels like a real girly indulgence but I think nails should be neatly manicured all the time and even just a coat of clear gloss can make all the difference. Wearing coloured nail polish can really alter your look and give your outfit an edge. I paint mine once a week and either have them done at a salon or do them myself at home. If they are painted well, your colour should last for a week. When I'm planning what polish colour to go for, I think about what I've got coming up in the week and if I've got lots of evening events, I often go for red because as well as being a classic colour, it's an instant mood lifter.

Like skin and hair, everyone has different types of nails. In the same way that our skin might be classed as dry, oily or sensitive, some people's nails are more brittle and prone to splitting or have oilier nail beds than others. If your nails are in bad condition, seek out a manicurist and ask their advice on what products might help.

THE DIY MANICURE

Having your finger or toenails manicured by a professional at a salon is a lovely treat but it is very easy to get to grips with giving yourself a basic manicure at home. Make sure you give yourself enough time to let the polish dry afterwards. I am definitely not patient when it comes to letting my nails dry but there is nothing more annoying than smudged nails!

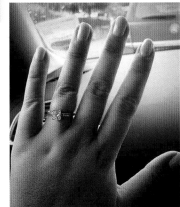

★ Position your tools and arms on a flat surface and start by removing any previously applied nail polish. An acetone-based nail-polish remover is a bit harsher than non-acetone removers, but the acetone removers get the job done faster.

★ Then clip your nails and gently file them (in one direction) into whatever shape you prefer. Most people opt for a gently round or square shape or somewhere in between. Finish by buffing the sides and tops of your nails to give you an even surface.

★ Ahh… and relax! Place your hands in a bowl of warm water and add some cleanser to gently clean, while you put your feet up for a few minutes. Dry your hands then soften the cuticle with oil and gently push the cuticles back.

★ Many people now trim their cuticles but there is a lot of room to go wrong and over-cutting is a bad idea because the cuticle helps to protect the nail bed from bacteria. Trim the free edges and be very gentle.

★ Exfoliate and moisturise your hands all over into the nails and cuticles and if you want, give yourself a lovely hand massage while you are doing it. Finish by swiping each nail with nail polish remover.

★ Paint the nail in coats, starting with the base coat, followed by two coats of colour and then a top coat to add shine. If you're new to painting your own nails use lighter shades of polish because mistakes are less noticeable.

★ Clean up any mistakes and voilà! Now wait for the polish to dry; I always find that getting immersed in an episode of one of my favourite TV shows is a good distraction!

MY TOP 10
NAIL TIPS

1 | **ALWAYS MOISTURISE**
Moisturise your hands and nails as much as the rest of your body, so you keep the skin hydrated and soft. This will also reduce hangnails, rough cuticles and brittle nails.

2 | **USE CUTICLE OIL**
Always use a cuticle oil to provide moisture for softer and supple cuticles. I also use it every night before I go to bed and keep it on my bedside table (with my Eight Hour Cream!) to remind myself.

3 | **HAVE A CLEAN SURFACE**
Always have a super-clean surface for painting. Any trace of dust or leftover polish will keep the new nail polish from sticking. The easiest thing to do is before painting, wipe nails with a cotton ball soaked in nail polish remover because this will also remove traces of any lotion.

4 | **REMEMBER YOUR BASE COAT AND TOP COAT**
Use a base coat to give the polish something to latch on to and, after painting, seal the colour with a slow-setting top coat. This will leave a harder, more protective finish so your colour will stay on for longer.

5 | **PAINT WITH CARE**
When applying your polish, do it with three narrow

and even strokes, one down the middle and one down each side of the nail. Then wait a few minutes and apply a second coat. Try to use sparingly; the thicker the layer of polish, the more likely it is to be uneven.

6 | EXPRESS YOUR INDIVIDUALITY
When it comes to colour for everyday wear, choose something that you like and which expresses how you are feeling – anything that makes you feel fabulous!

7 | KEEP NAILS STRONG
Avoid filing nails as soon as you get out of the shower because they will be more susceptible to breaking.

8 | FOR TOES TOO
All the tips for manicures apply to pedicures. Remember to pay close attention to your tootsies and give yourself a regular DIY pedicure.

9 | USE GLOVES
After a manicure, always wear rubber gloves to do the washing up because soapy suds will wreak havoc on your beautiful nails.

10 | STORE WELL
Always store your nail polishes in a cool, dry place and away from sunlight, as this can leave them discoloured. If you can, keep the bottles stored in an upright position because if they lie sideways it is harder to shake the pigments back together.

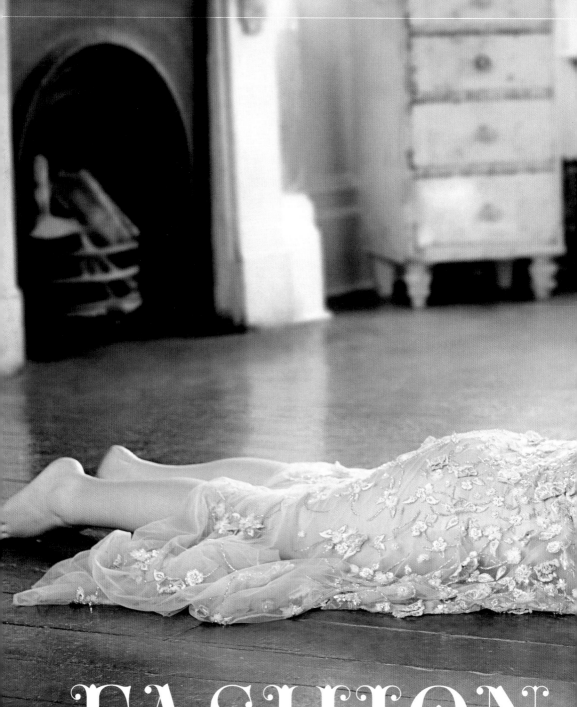

FASHION

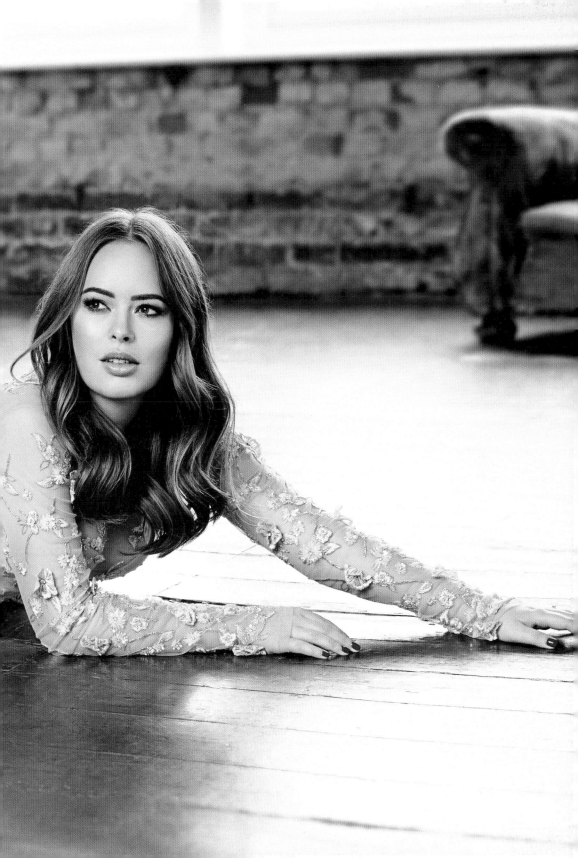

I've always loved dressing up. I think there is something really wonderful about being able to grab a few items from your wardrobe, put them on, stand in front of the mirror and feel like a completely new person. Fashion is a great way of expressing our personalities and using our imaginations. Personally, I find myself really inspired by girls and women walking down the street. Rather than stare at good-looking guys as they wander past, Jim is always pointing out that I am always studying girls! I'm never afraid to ask where someone bought their skirt, shoes or coat, so can often be found chasing after unsuspecting girls. Living in London, the fashions are so eclectic and so many people have such great style. In fact, I would be very happy just to sit with a Starbucks latte and people-watch for hours!

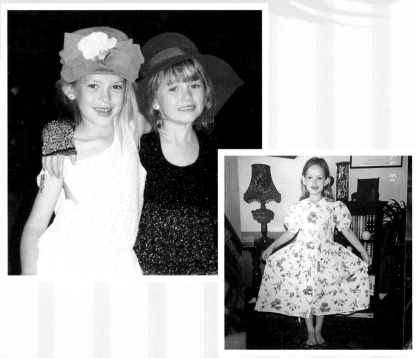

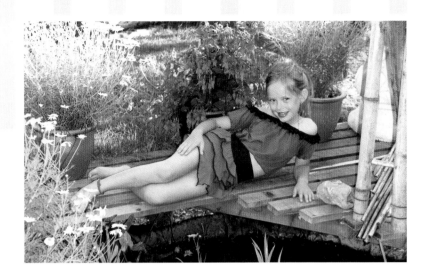

Dad made me a pretty pink cotton dress when I was one and my love of fashion just snowballed from there. I adored all the items he would bring back from car boot sales and I loved the constant dressing up. I even insisted on having my ears pierced when I was five! Mum felt so bad about it, my dad took me to have them done. I took great pleasure in trying on my mum's wedding dress and her shoes and apparently I always used to notice what family and friends were wearing and if they had new outfits on.

I've never really stuck to the rules. Growing up, my dad did a lot of gardening and we would all help out, including the children my mum looked after and, like now, style always won over practicality. I remember one digging session, where I styled myself with a cute little handbag and a floppy 70s hat for the occasion! Mum says a lot of my clothes when I was little were hand-me-downs from friends and cousins and I would often end up with quite a few party dresses because they were always in good condition. As a child I always loved getting dressed and used to change my outfit ten times a day. Another favourite pastime when I was small was dressing up all my friends and then making them parade down the stairs, like it was the catwalk, while I commentated on the clothes they were wearing.

When I was a teenager, I loved being able to buy my own clothes. My job at Starbucks really came about because I always wanted the latest things. Starbucks was right next to Topshop and I used to go there on my lunch break and try things on. I could only put things on hold for three days, but I used to keep putting whatever it was back on hold again and again until payday when I would rush in and pick the items up. If I saw something I really loved, I would work every shift I could so I could afford to buy it!

There have been a few personal fashion highlights from the past few years. I never normally work with stylists but in the last couple of years, I have been lucky enough to be dressed by some designers. Last year Burberry dressed me for the *Noah* premiere, which was a dream come true. I worked with one of their top stylists, Kay Ganesh, who helped me to step out of my comfort zone, and I wore a stunning sky-blue satin-backed crêpe dress. I have also done a shoot with Mulberry, when they have dressed me and Jim and I starred in a 'A Day In The Life Feature' for Mulberry.com. Going to London Fashion Week is always

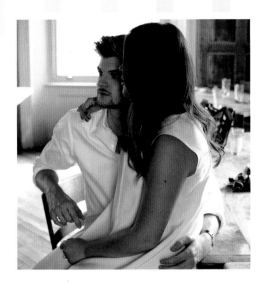
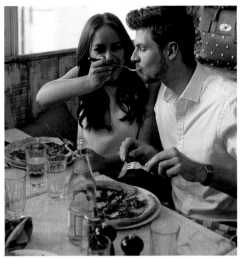

such a brilliant experience and has given me a real insight into the world of designer fashion in general. As well as seeing the latest fashions being modelled on the catwalk, I love looking at what the guests are wearing, who is sitting on the front row and how they mix pieces together.

Sometimes it can be quite nerve-wracking if I'm sitting on the front row because I know that other people will be examining what I'm wearing, but I think I've got braver and more experimental with my choices more recently. I've started having more fun and taking risks.

While I'm passionate about clothes, I don't consider myself a fashion expert, but since my YouTube videos have become more popular and I've got more involved with fashion brands, I feel like I'm learning more and more and hope to share some of what I have picked up with you.

DRESSING FOR YOUR BODY TYPE

Fashion is all about dressing for your body. If you know your body type, then you should be able to find clothes that flatter your shape and look fabulous. Body shape is all about proportion and helping to make your proportions look their very best. Never focus on height or weight but instead think about shape and silhouette. This is crucial for self-confidence. Knowing you have chosen clothes that showcase your body in the best possible light, you can relax and enjoy yourself!

I didn't realise that I had a waist until three years ago. I just thought I had chubby legs and short arms, while my friends had gorgeous long slim arms and legs. My staple outfit was big jumpers and Topshop skinny jeans and if I wanted a slightly smarter look, I would buy slightly more expensive jumpers! I hated having full-length pictures taken and never felt particularly comfortable with my choices. But I would never leave the house in this outfit these days because I now know it doesn't flatter my shape at all. It was a trip to see a personal shopper that made me realise what clothes suited my hourglass shape best, like pretty dresses with nipped-in waists and high-waisted skirts that showed off my narrowest point and skimmed across my hips and thighs. By wearing clothes that hugged my figure and my waist, I looked like I had a lost a stone.

Each one of us is unique and our bodies are too, but the main categories I'm going to cover are petite, pear, apple, hourglass and rectangle. You might clearly be one shape

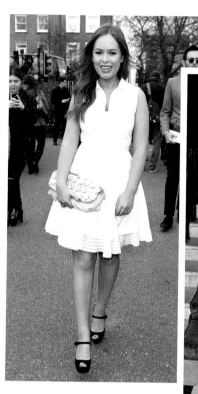

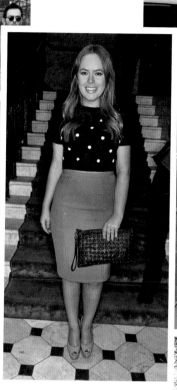

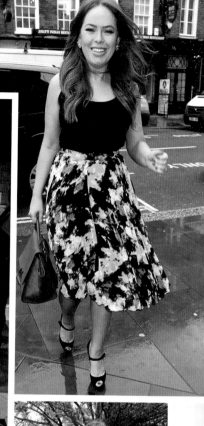

or you might be a blend of two or more categories. I'm a blend of pear and hourglass.

One way of finding ideas for how to dress for your shape is to find a celebrity, or someone who inspires you, who has a similar shape to you. See what they are wearing and what styles of clothes you think look good on them and then study your own wardrobe to see if you have anything similar.

PEAR

You have a pear-shape if your lower body is wider than your upper body, so if your hips are wider than your shoulders, you fall into this category.

★ Accentuate your top half with pretty patterned tops or by wearing a statement necklace.

★ In winter, make use of jackets. A longer jacket that ends past the hip will give the impression of a long, lean line.

★ Choose heavier materials that flatter and streamline your shape.

★ Plunging necklines will help to elongate your upper body and draw attention upwards.

HOURGLASS

Hourglass girls are known for their curves and have bigger boobs and bottoms but much slimmer waists.

★ Wear well fitting underwear because this will give you the best support and accentuate your curves to the max.

★ Always choose fitted clothing. Since hourglass girls have well-defined waists, draw attention to this feature with a belt, high-waisted skirt, or top or jacket with a fitted waist.

★ Avoid baggy or boxy clothing (like I used to wear) because this will just hide your curvy shape and little waist. Show your figure off to the max!

★ Choose lightweight fabrics like cotton and silk because they tend to glide over your curves and flatter your shape.

★ Low, slimming necklines will be most flattering and will balance out your figure.

APPLE

An apple-shaped girl's best assets are her legs. She will have a small bottom and more weight around her torso and arms.

★ Keep the clothing line straight to slightly fitted but wear soft and lightweight fabrics, to avoid unnecessary bulk around your top half.

★ To draw attention to your legs and bum, wear shorter clothing on the bottom half and keep to bright and light colours on your lower body.

★ High-waisted skirts and trousers will give the appearance of a waist, as will tops that are wraparounds or have ruching or a tie around the waist.

★ Avoid high necklaces because they can make your upper body appear even more out of proportion.

★ Choose single-breasted or V-neck jackets to give the illusion of a smaller, longer upper body.

PETITE

Petite girls are little more than five feet and have smaller proportions than average.

★ Avoid wearing tops with horizontal lines because they tend to make you look wider and shorter than you really are. Large patterns can also be overpowering. Instead, choose clothes with vertical stripes, vertical seams, vertical pleats, and long lapels to help elongate your shape and make you appear taller.

★ Choose tops with three-quarter length sleeves and V or scoop necklines to help elongate your silhouette.

★ The easiest way to add height is by wearing a heel, but avoid any with ankle straps because these will thicken your legs and make you appear short.

★ Avoid oversized bags or accessories because these will overwhelm your petite frame.

★ Monochrome looks are great for petite girls because they help elongate your appearance.

RECTANGLE

Rectangle girls have waist, hip and shoulder widths which are similar and are usually on the slim side. Slender rectangles tend to look quite athletic.

★ Softly structured jackets can gently shape the waist and coats that belt at the waist have the same affect.

★ Use strong blocks of colour to help define your features.

★ Layering adds more dimension and definition to a simple rectangle body shape.

★ It's essential to have good-fitting underwear because this will make the most of the curves you have.

★ Almost all kinds of trousers will look good on you, except boyfriend-style or baggy jeans.

WHERE TO SHOP

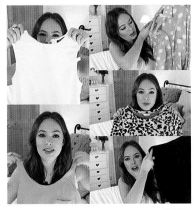

Starting with the high street, where the brands are simply amazing; I have always bought my clothes from high street shops like Topshop, Miss Selfridge, River Island and French Connection. I build my wardrobe around great high street staples, such as trousers, skirts, dresses and jumpers, and then throw in the odd designer item or pair of shoes to mix up my look. The high street is great for so many things: Topshop is fab for most stuff, River Island does brilliant jeans that never lose their shape and last for ages, Primark is great for vest tops, and I find Zara is the best place to go if I'm looking for individual items. It's worth noting that there are always designer imitations on the high street, so if you see something you love on the catwalk or being worn by a celebrity, it will invariably turn up on the high street ten times cheaper fairly quickly. Often designers pair up with high street stores and some recent collaborations include Alexander Wang for H&M, Marques' Almeida for Topshop and Mary Katrantzou for adidas. Sometimes these collections contain some real gems.

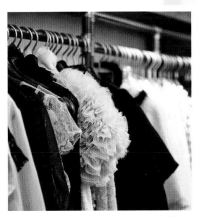

I've also found some great items at supermarkets' clothing concessions and they have clearly upped their game over the past few years. Don't always think that because something is cheap that it won't look good.

I think you can pick up some real bargains at the supermarket and because you're not spending a fortune, if you wear something just a few times, there is no need to feel guilty! Last summer I had a smock denim dress from George at Asda that I lived in. The quality of this dress felt great and I washed it every other day and it kept its colour and shape. All my favourite pyjamas come from F&F at Tesco.

I also love shopping online at sites like ASOS. If I have a free day at home and I'm really exhausted and lying on the sofa with a mug of tea, I love browsing online. On many online shopping sites, once you've ordered over a certain amount, most of the time delivery is free and so are returns, so if you find shopping stressful or hate getting undressed in changing rooms, this is a great option. It also means there is no queuing, no massive shopping bags and no sore feet! Just don't do what I do sometimes and go impulse shopping and then have a big surprise when it all turns up and you have to send it back!

The other place I shop is in vintage or charity shops. I really got into shopping for older items when I was about sixteen and I found that I could pick up some really interesting vintage jewellery, leather bags and shoes that had barely been worn for hardly anything. One of my favourite looks was pairing second-hand floral granny skirts with belts and a Topshop white T-shirt. Sometimes these shops are packed to the brim and can feel a bit overwhelming but my advice is to not feel intimidated. The best tactic is to get stuck in; you can really uncover some treasures if you look carefully enough. It's also great to customise items from charity shops or learn to mix and match with old clothes, because they are normally really cheap and even if you only wear them a few times it doesn't matter. Also, another big bonus when you wear vintage clothing is that you know no one will be wearing the same outfit as you!

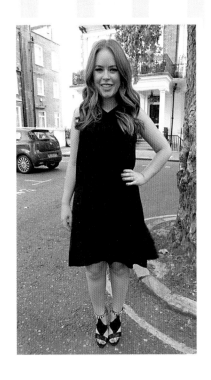

It's only been far more recently that I've been able to treat myself to the odd designer outfit and if I think I'm going to use something a lot then it's OK to spend a bit more. If you are buying designer items, look for things that are relatively timeless and won't go out of style. One of my favourite designer pieces is a black dress I bought last year from Sportmax, which I love because the material is so thick and silky, it just hangs beautifully and is so flattering. Although it's not like the shape I normally go for, it is really simple and chic. I wore it to the *Guardians of the Galaxy* premiere and I just know I will wear it for many years to come.

There are great websites where you can borrow designer items for a fraction of the cost of the real thing and I used to do this a lot. All the sites work slightly differently, but the one I signed up to allowed you to pick three options and a back-up size and only pay for the one you chose.

I have worn a couple of Hervé Leger dresses, and the Tibi dress that I wore for my first Tanya Burr Cosmetics launch came via those sites – mine for a few days only!

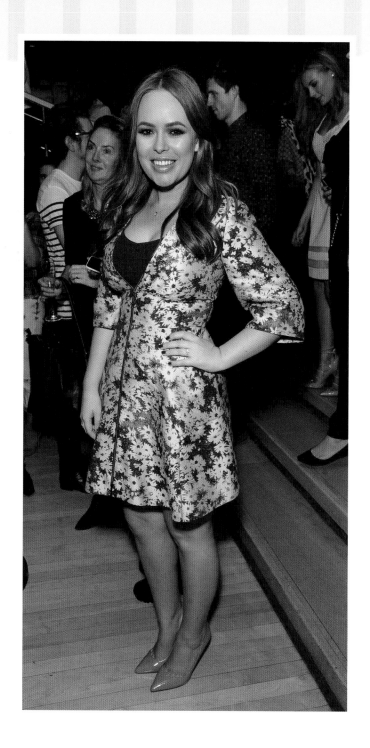

At the moment one of the designers I really admire is Stella McCartney. If I see someone in a magazine or on the red carpet and like their outfit, a lot of the time they have been dressed by her. I wore a Stella McCartney dress to my lashes launch last year and it felt really special. I also love Mulberry. Their clothes are so classic and quintessentially British. The quality is always amazing and my Mulberry handbag was my first-ever designer handbag, so it holds a special place in my heart!

HOW TO ACCESSORISE

Accessories can really personalise your outfit and often shoes and bags last for decades – much longer than clothes! The great thing about accessories is that they can really change an outfit and make your look rockier, more classic or sexier. However, it's important to know when to stop. I think one or two well-chosen items can really lift a look but don't go overboard. For example, when wearing a statement necklace, I pair it with simple studs rather than big dangly earrings. If you want to wear lots of bracelets, don't wear too much around the neck. You don't have to match your bag, shoes and belt either. It's all about getting an even balance for a polished look.

SHOES

Shoes are probably most girls' number one accessory. When it comes to building a shoe collection, don't feel like you need to have everything straight away. I finally feel like I have covered all bases with my shoe collection, so any more are just a bonus! It depends on your style what you think your key items are, but for me I wanted some nude pointed high heels, some nude peep-toe high heels, some black high heels, some black peep-toe high heels, an intricate and ornate high heel, some tan wedges, some black wedges, ankle boots with a heel, flat ankle boots, loafers, gladiator sandals and ballet flats. You can buy very good shoes on the high street from shops like Kurt Geiger, who do beautiful classics, and River Island, where they do some quite innovative designs and so look slightly more designer.

Just like accessories, shoes can really change a look. While high heels add glamour and poise to an outfit, wedges are a great alternative because they are comfortable and practical and look great with summer dresses. They are perfect if you are going to an event where stilettos aren't quite right but you still want to wear a heel.

Last year, I lived in a pair of black leather gladiator sandals all summer. I always think black leather looks quite cool and I love really strappy sandals. I like to buy gladiator sandals with a slight wedge because it is slightly more flattering and stops me from looking flat-footed. With loafers, they are like blazers and can really smarten up an outfit. I love wearing a cool skater dress with a pair of loafers because it gives the look a slightly masculine edge.

JEWELLERY

When it comes to jewellery, statement pieces get me really excited because I think they can take your outfit to the next level. They are such an easy way to dress up a simple outfit, like a plain dress or T-shirt and jeans. For example, a casual graphic tee becomes dressier when you pair it with a glam sparkly statement necklace, while a neon necklace with a grey tee can bring an awesome twist of colour to your look. I do like delicate jewellery and wear a plain diamond necklace, which Jim bought me, as an everyday piece, and I also like sparkly studs because I find that they reflect the light on your face. However, for me, when it comes to big events and dressing up, statement items are key. I don't think you need to spend a lot on statement jewellery; as well as shopping on the high street, street markets and charity shops can produce real finds. One of my favourite statement rings is from Portobello market.

HATS

I need to give hats a special mention because I am a big fan of mine. I wear fedoras all year round and as well as a

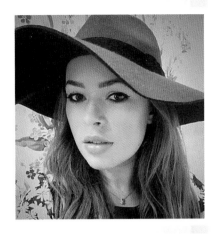

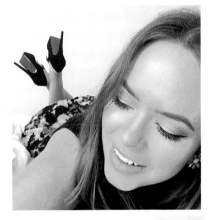

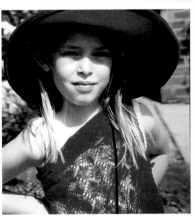

black one, I wear a mauve-coloured one in the summer. I don't think hats are for everybody, but this can be the one accessory that sets you apart, whether you're at a formal event or just running to the shops to buy milk. I don't tend to wear scarves all year round because I think they add too much volume to my chest, but when it's really cold, I love to wrap up with a tartan scarf over my winter coat and a woolly hat for a really cute look.

BAGS

Finally… bags! I've always been into handbags and love changing up my bag. I can't pretend my bags are tidy and organised – they are super-messy – but I have perfected the art of not taking my whole bedroom with me. Some girls like to have one everyday bag that they use until it breaks but I like having a range of colours for different occasions or to complement various outfits. At the moment, I have a thing about electric-blue bags and I think they can look fabulous paired with jeans and a white T-shirt. My favourite bags are ones you can carry in different ways. One tip I've learned is that if you have a gorgeous leather handbag, store it in a dust bag with tissue paper inside so it keeps its shape. The same applies to shoes: I like to keep them in their original boxes and stick Polaroids on the outside, so I can locate my favourite pairs.

WHAT'S IN MY BAG?

★ My keys on my red heart-shaped Smythson key ring: my parents bought me this key ring for Christmas one year. I think Smythson is a gorgeous brand.

★ A book: I am often on a train or plane, so I always make sure I have my latest book with me.

★ Mints: I hate the look of chewing gum, so always carry mints to freshen my breath. Recently I was at Zoe's house chewing gum while editing my vlog – it looked gross!

★ My Prada wallet: I bought this bright-red leather, girly wallet in Prada when I visited New York with Jim the first time. It's really structured and has a pretty bow with gold trimmings on the front. Inside I keep my money, cards and some old Polaroid pictures of Jim and me messing around.

★ Sunglasses: my favourite sunnies are my mirrored Ray-Bans for everyday or my big Prada sunglasses for a more glam look. I'm quite good about looking after mine but if you find you leave them all over the place, then the high street do fantastic on-style sunglasses.

★ A small make-up bag: there is no point carrying a big make-up bag around and I just carry the items that I might need to do touch-ups. I carry a lipstick, lip balm, lip gloss, a powder, a powder brush and a concealer.

★ My iPhone

★ My Oyster/travel card

★ Earphones

★ Ear cuff: if I want to make an outfit look interesting, I can just add my ear cuff from Urban Outfitters, which makes it look like I have loads of piercings up the side of my ear.

★ Some hairclips: if my hair is getting in my face, I take two bits from either side, twirl them around and clip them onto either side or I use them to make a ponytail look more interesting.

★ Hand sanitiser

HOW TO ORGANISE YOUR WARDROBE

Twice a year I like to clear my wardrobe to see what I have and clean out all the dusty corners at the back. It's really useful for unearthing clothes that you haven't worn in ages but want to wear more. A good time to do this is between seasons, like from winter to spring or summer to autumn, when you might be putting clothes away or be thinking about buying some new items for the next season.

★ Start by getting into something easy to wear and if you have long hair, tie it back so it doesn't get in the way.

★ Tidy up the area around your wardrobe, so you've got surfaces to put your clothes out. I also find this gets me in the mood for cleaning and clears my head a bit.

★ Take everything out of your wardrobe – yes everything! – and as you do, put each item into one of four piles: keep, store, donate to the charity shop, and bin. The bin pile should contain clothes that are unwearable and have holes or are stained; the things you wouldn't even give to a charity shop. The donate pile should contain wearable clothes but ones that you know you no longer want, to go to friends for a root through or the charity shop. The keep pile will go back in the wardrobe, so these are the things you one hundred per cent want to keep, and the store pile is for clothes that are seasonally inappropriate but which you want to keep for next year. For example, in spring you'll probably want to put away thick winter coats and jumpers.

★ There are lots of ways to store clothes between seasons but I find the most useful way is to use vacuum-packed clear bags. They are ideal for storing bulky items and great because you can see what you have stored when it comes to unpacking. I tend to store these at the top of my wardrobe, under my bed – or anywhere I can find space!

★ When I go through my pile of clothes to keep, I double-check I definitely want to keep them by trying the items on or asking Jim. I find taking photos is quite useful to see what I look like. If you've not worn something for a year, it's normally a sign that it needs to go into your donate pile. Maybe it doesn't fit or is a trend that has gone out of fashion. Put the things you are unsure about in a maybe pile, put it away in a clear bag and set a reminder on your phone for a couple of months' time. If you haven't thought about the clothes, then they do need to be added to the donate bag.

★ Now give your wardrobe a thorough clean with a cloth and cleaning spray. If your wardrobe is anything like mine, there will be a lot of dust. Don't forget to do the drawers and surrounding areas!

★ Now return your clothes to your wardrobe, one item at a time. Everyone has a different way of organising their wardrobes and it might be time to replan yours. Some people like to colour code their wardrobe but my personal way is to put different items together, so smart dresses, day dresses, jumpers, shirts etc. in separate groups.

★ Always try to hang as much as possible because it makes it much easier to see what you have. Then you can see if there are any gaps in your wardrobe and things that you might need to pick up, stuff that you have lusted after or think might work well with your current clothes.

★ Hopefully now you will have a streamlined, de-cluttered and clean-smelling wardrobe (and maybe a shopping list!).

MY TOP 10
FASHION TIPS

1 | **DON'T ALWAYS FEEL PRESSURISED TO FOLLOW THE TRENDS**
Fashion trends are constantly changing and while something might be really in fashion, it might not always suit you. Recently, there was a trend for 1950s'-style dresses and I loved it because they really suit my hourglass shape and nipped-in waist, while covering my bum and thighs. Equally (sorry if I'm contradicting myself!), if you adore a trend and think it's really cool and just want to wear it, go for it.

2 | **HAVE A NICE SILHOUETTE**
Dressing to flatter your figure is a key rule to looking stylish, so always aim for your clothes to have a pretty silhouette, with clean lines.

3 | **IF YOU LOVE SOMETHING JUST WEAR IT**
Style is so personal, so if you have an item in a crazy colour or a piece of mad costume jewellery that you love, then just wear it. Fashion is all about having fun.

4 | **INVEST IN PIECES YOU'LL WEAR A LOT**
Build your wardrobe around great timeless staples that you know will pay for themselves over and over again. If you wear jeans a lot, then splash out on the perfect, most flattering pair or if you're choosing a bag you plan to use every day, look for something leather as it will last longer.

5 | BOOK A PERSONAL SHOPPER

Personal shoppers are amazing and are sometimes offered free in department stores and big flagship shops. Jim's mum used to be a personal shopper and I know she helped so many women – including me – with their style. Personal shoppers encourage you to try on things you normally wouldn't pick and can show you what suits your figure best. If you're going for the experience and there is no minimum spend, don't feel pressured to buy something. If you feel awkward, tell them that you want to go away and think about it.

6 | TAKE PHOTOS

One of my top tips is that when you go shopping take a friend with you and get them to take pictures of you in every outfit you try on. If I'm on my own it's much harder because taking pictures in the mirror doesn't really work. Don't pose for the photo, just look natural and make sure you look the same in each one. After a big shopping session, I go for lunch with my friend and flick through all the photos and it becomes so clear what looks good and what doesn't because you can compare your looks.

7 | PLAN WHAT YOU'RE GOING TO WEAR

If you have a big party or event on, plan what you are going to wear in advance or you'll end up with a serious case of 'floordrobe', with everything flung on the floor, and feel really flustered and stressed. When I'm invited to a big event I start thinking almost immediately about what I could wear, so I have lots of time to plan.

8 | GET CLOTHES TAILORED OR CUSTOMISED

If something doesn't fit properly and you're not a whizz with a needle and thread yourself, don't be afraid to use a tailor. I have a slim waist and wider hips, which means often things are baggy around my middle, so I tailor a lot of my clothes. Recently I bought a Topshop skirt that I loved but it didn't fit very well, so I took it to a local tailor. When she had finished with it, not only did it fit perfectly, it looked like a designer item! Customising your clothes can also be a way to have fun and express your creativity. It can range from simple ideas, like changing the buttons on a cardigan, to something more ambitious, such as changing a pair of jeans into denim shorts.

9 | RESTYLE ITEMS

Skip an expensive shopping spree by restyling your clothes. Mix and match different items together or wear them with different shoes and accessories to achieve a completely different look.

10 | THINK ABOUT THE SMALL DETAILS

I always find accessories to incorporate into my look when getting dressed because it's the small details that can complete an outfit. Whether it's an amazing ring, a cool pair of shoes or a skinny belt, having accessories can make all the difference.

A final tip... Accept your shape and embrace it. Everyone has something great about their figure and so whatever yours is, show it off!

NOTES

List your favourite fashion items...

$\heartsuit$

MY TOP 10
FAVOURITE ITEMS

1 | **NEEDLE & THREAD EMBELLISHED BLOSSOM DRESS**

This is a burgundy mini-dress, with a sheer cover embellished with jewels and a skinny belt, which nips me in at the waist. I bought it online from ASOS because it caught my eye and I thought it looked pretty. When it arrived, I completely fell in love with it.

2 | **SMART BURBERRY COAT**

This is a classic black cashmere–wool mix coat, a real investment item. It's single-breasted and comes down to just above the knee. It fits perfectly, feels gorgeous and smartens up any outfit.

3 | **AMERICAN APPAREL RIDING PANTS**

These are classic high-waisted trousers, which do up with buttons and a zip so they never fall down. I find them so much more flattering than jeans or leggings and they last ages. They are an everyday staple for me, rather than jeans, which I like on other people but not on me. I also really like the American Apparel Disco Pants and they are also really slimming but they are in shiny latex, so can make your legs look quite big in photos.

4 | **REISS BLACK BLAZER**

My Reiss black blazer is really easy to wear and looks great with almost anything. I find some blazers really drown me because I am quite petite but this one is cropped, with three-quarter-length sleeves, which is perfect for my body shape. Even with biker boots or leggings and high heels, it looks great.

5 | REISS FEDORA HAT

I think a hat gives my outfit a bit of an edge. I particularly like wearing my fedora with pretty dresses; I think it is a really cute look.

6 | CHRISTIAN LOUBOUTIN SHOES

I have two pairs of super-high peep-toe Louboutins, one in black and one in nude. My first pair, the black ones, were a present from Jim a couple of Christmases ago. I would always look them up online but I didn't tell Jim I wanted them, so I don't know how he knew. I had opened all my presents at my parents' house and then we went to his mum's and he pointed out that there was another one for me. I saw that it had his writing on it and I was really confused. As soon as I opened it, saw the box and lifted the tissue paper – and saw they were Louboutins, I cried!

7 | BIKER-STYLE ANKLE BOOTS

I'm too passionate about fashion to always go with a comfy shoe at special events, but for everyday wear, these boots are so comfy. They also give a tough edge to any outfit.

8 | MULBERRY CARA BAG
This is my everyday bag and it's great that I can wear it as a rucksack, on my shoulder or use it as a tote. It's the Taupe Silky Classic Calf and I'm a big fan of the colour and the lion rivets, which make it unique and special.

9 | AQUASCUTUM TRENCH COAT
Last year I went on the hunt for the perfect trench coat. I wanted a very specific length that didn't come below my knee but ended at the mid-thigh. Jim and I spent the whole day walking up and down Oxford Street and Regent Street. We ended up splitting up and he went into Aquascutum and I went into Banana Republic, then he called and told me he had found 'The One'. It's the best spring coat.

10 | VERY.CO.UK HIGH-WAISTED LEATHER SKIRT
In September last year I was lucky enough to be asked to curate my own clothing collection for Very.co.uk and I got this skirt. It is cool as it's mid-length, so a bit different

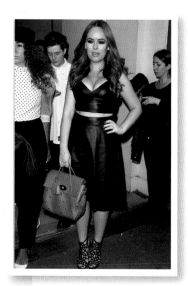

to anything else in my wardrobe, and because it's leather it's quite a statement piece. I wore it to a London Fashion Week event and again at Amity Fest.

NOTES

List the celebrities whose style you admire and why...

♡

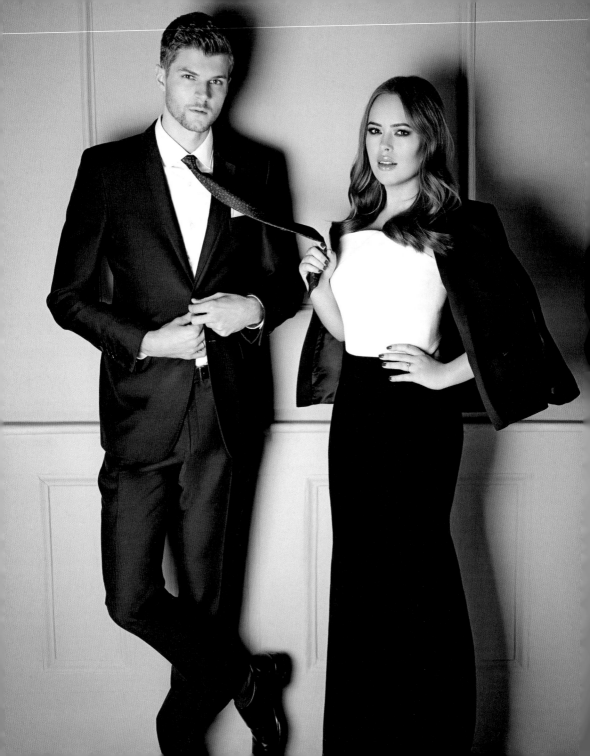

LOVE

'There are dreamers and there are realists in this world, you think the dreamers would find the dreamers and the realists would find the realists, but more often than not the opposite is true. See, the dreamers need the realists to keep the dreamers from soaring too close to the sun. And the realists? Well, without the dreamers, they might not ever get off the ground.'

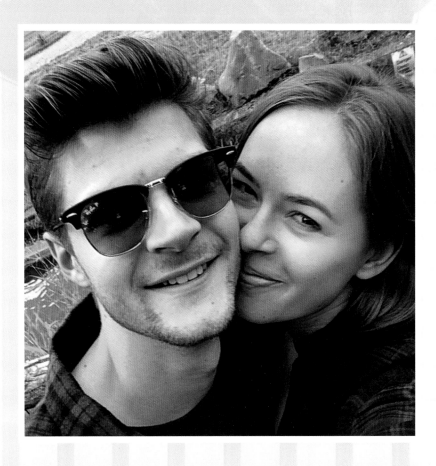

I love this cute quote from *Modern Family* because I think it really sums up my relationship with Jim. We joke that we are just like the characters Cam and Mitch and this quote makes me well up every time I hear it. I am such a dreamer and think I can do whatever I want and anything can happen, whereas Jim is such a realist. He might have ideas for things but he immediately pushes them out of his head. I love the fact that we bring out the best in each other. Jim is just one of the best people that I know; he is so gentlemanly, honest and kind. We never freak out about the same things; we balance each other out perfectly. When we first got together, I was seventeen and Jim was eighteen and people told us that we were too young and it would never last, but from the early days I knew it would because he's just the best.

Before I met Jim, I hadn't had a proper relationship but since the age of eleven, I'd always had boyfriends. I remember going out with my first boyfriend in high school. We used to hang out together and hold hands at lunchtime but it was totally not serious. My first kiss happened one lunchtime, when everyone was telling us we should kiss and we did. I had no idea how to kiss someone; I hadn't practised on my hand or anything like that, like some girls do. I didn't have a clue! All I remember was that I kept my eyes open and it went on forever. One of my friends came up to me afterwards and she said, 'Tan, you know when you kiss a boy you need to make sure you shut your eyes?' She had clearly seen it happen. It's so awkward and cringey remembering that! Those romances at school were quite funny because one day you would be going out with a boy and the next day you wouldn't be and he would be going out with your friend instead. I never really went on proper dates before I met Jim; it was more casual, where we would go around to each other's houses or just hang out in groups of friends.

As I mentioned earlier, Jim and I met at a house party and we swapped numbers. We had had a great evening and I enjoyed his company but I didn't think anything more about it. The next day I had a shift in Starbucks. He had told his best friend that he really liked me, so his friend literally pushed him into the shop where I was working in an attempt to force him to come and talk to me. Jim panicked because he had never been into Starbucks as he doesn't like coffee, but he ordered one and went to sit in the upstairs seating area. Rather than drinking the coffee, he spent the whole time nervously chewing on one of the wooden sticks they give you to mix your drink! Luckily, I was on washing-up duty, which meant I could go upstairs to collect the cups and say hello to him. Jim always says that he was rubbish with girls and would say the wrong things, but we had a good chat and he offered to wait for me to finish my shift so we could hang out afterwards.

After work, he met me and we went and stood around the nearby ice rink and watched the skaters and just chatted. Afterwards, he walked me to my bus stop and I got the bus home. He was a real gentleman and very sweet but I didn't know it would develop into anything.

For the first week or so, we were definitely just friends. We hung out casually a few more times and, once or twice, he met me on my lunch break because he was working at an indie clothing shop called Elements nearby. If we couldn't coordinate our lunch breaks, I would go and see him in the shop when I had my break and Jim would come into Starbucks where I would be told off for talking to him all the time when I was supposed to be washing the dishes or making coffees!

When my friend Kate asked me what I thought of him, I was unsure. I had always been attracted to the bad boys or naughty boys at school and college and I had never gone out with a guy so lovely as Jim before. Kate said she thought he was just gorgeous – both to look at and the way he looked after me, and Kate too if she was with us. By that point, we were texting all the time and it got to the point when I was really excited to get his texts, so I knew that I was starting to develop feelings for him. When my phone buzzed I would be really happy and show my friends all the texts he had sent. I loved the fact that Jim never messed around, unlike other boys I had been on dates with or texted who wanted to play it really cool the whole time. He was never over-the-top but I knew from the start that he liked me. However, he had a

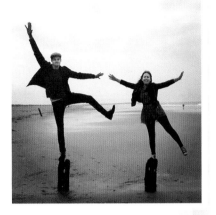

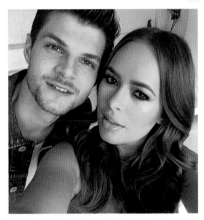

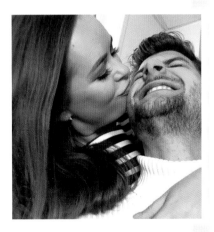

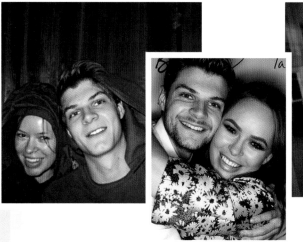

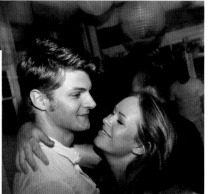

dodgy phone that sent every text twice – so he actually seemed a lot more keen than he had intended! It was so funny when I told him and he was mortified! We still laugh about it now.

Our first official date was to the cinema to see *The Holiday* with Jude Law, Kate Winslet, Jack Black and Cameron Diaz. I remember that he sat next to me with his feet up on the chair in front. He seemed nervous! He's since said that he couldn't concentrate on the film at all because he was wondering whether we should be talking or if he should hold my hand. I was completely oblivious and really got into the film and loved it. When the film finished, he walked me to my bus stop again and as the bus pulled up, I was waiting for him to kiss me, but I knew he wasn't going to because he was shy, so I kissed him. I was wearing flat shoes and he is so much taller than me that I literally had to jump up off the pavement! I don't think we said we were officially going out but it was after that date that I think we knew we were an item.

We fell in love really quickly. At that time, I was still at school studying for my A-Levels and Jim was at uni doing his degree. We both worked every weekend but in our free time we used to go to the cinema, eat out at Pizza Express and just hang out together. I remember that pretty early on I made him watch the whole *OC* box set from start to finish because I didn't think I could go out with someone who didn't know who Marissa, Seth and Ryan were. He claims he hated it but I think he enjoyed some bits! He was still nervous around me for a while and never wanted to eat in front of me, so we watched the box set with no food or drink for six hours!

Once I tried to impress him by taking a PlayStation game called Burnout to his house and claimed I was really good at it but I wasn't at all. We used to spend a lot of time in his house and get takeaways with his family. Neither of us drove and because he lived in town, it was much more convenient for going to school and work.

After leaving school, I spent all my time at his house and after eight months, I eventually moved in. It was Jim who suggested I bring some more things to the house and use it as my base. Jim's mum Judy is great. She's really laidback and I loved being with his family. Eventually we lived at the house together for four years. When we could afford to move out, we decided to take the plunge. We really needed the space, because we used one room to film our videos, sleep in and for Jim to do his uni work in. We originally thought we'd try and buy somewhere but we worked out it would take us too much time to save for a deposit so decided to rent our own place together as a first step. We chose a converted barn in the middle of the countryside nearby. I think it was my idea because my friend Kate's family home is a barn conversion and I have so many fantastic memories of being there. It was the first time that either of us had bought loads of furniture. We spent so much time bargain hunting for things like sofas, a bed and a washing machine. Our biggest tip when it comes to furniture shopping is to never buy things full price – Jim's mum taught him that, because Jim has a twin, John, and because she always had to buy everything twice when they were growing up, she always asked for discounts. We bought most of our stuff for less than half price and our sofa was an absolute bargain.

We moved into the barn and experimented with it for a while but we weren't really that happy there. The barn was lovely but it wasn't very practical and although we both drove and had a car that we shared, I don't think we realised how much we loved being in town, where we could walk to the shops or order food really easily. It also had rubbish Wi-Fi and phone signal, which made work difficult. After a year we moved out of the barn and bought our first house together not far from Jim's family home near the centre of Norwich. We instantly loved it and really enjoyed our time together there.

We're not a very fiery couple and don't argue much at all. People told us that we would argue loads when we went on our three-month trip to Thailand and Australia, but if anything, we argued less than ever before. He looked out for me the whole time and would have his eye on me constantly to check I was OK. As part of our trip, we went on a sixteen-hour sleeper train from central Thailand to northern Thailand; the train carriage was filthy and tiny and there were disgusting cockroaches everywhere. The bunk beds were so narrow and had just enough space for one person, but I was too scared to sleep on my own, so Jim let me share his bunk, which wasn't very comfortable but very sweet of him!

We had some fairly bad luck when we were travelling and I was so happy I was with Jim. We went from Bangkok to the island Koh Samui but when we arrived late one evening, there were no tourists around; it was like they knew something that we didn't! It was raining gently but nothing could've prepared us for what lay ahead. The next morning we woke up to torrential rain and ended up getting trapped in the worst floods the island had seen for ten years. It was quite scary because we were staying in little huts just off the beach and the floods were so bad water was all over our floor and there was no power to charge our phones and let our families know that we were OK. There was only one luxury restaurant, which had a generator, so we went out and had

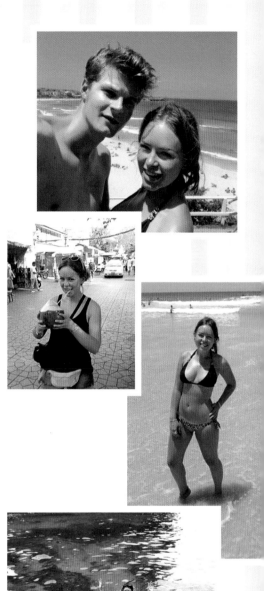

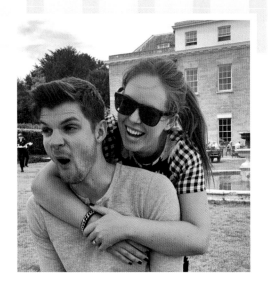
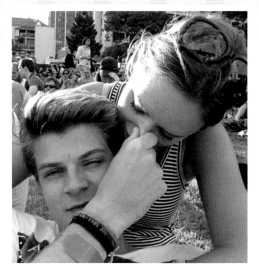

the only expensive meal of our entire travels. I was quite scared but Jim is so calm in situations like that. We slept that night with our rucksacks on our bed with us, and the following morning found we couldn't buy any breakfast because no food was able to get to the island. In the end, we got a trip back to the airport in this minibus that could barely make its way through the water. We eventually stayed at the airport and got a flight back to Bangkok. Jim was such a rock throughout the entire experience.

By the time we had been together for a few years, we each knew that the other person was 'The One'. We were so happy together. When I first watched *Twilight* and saw the relationship between Bella and Edward, I felt like they were a couple that loved each other in the same way that I love Jim! We never really had the, 'Shall we get married?' talk; it was more the case that one day when we were walking past a jewellers in Norwich, there were loads of sparkly rings in the window and I went to have a look at them. Then Jim started asking me about what type of ring I would like. It was just a bit of fun; I would try rings on in some of the jewellers and we decided which shop was our favourite.

When we went to New York in December 2012, I had a feeling he might propose but when we arrived Jim was acting so normal. I'm such a planner and will book all our trips and where we are going to eat wherever we go, but while Jim might say he wants to do something, he never plans. I had wondered if he might propose but after a couple of days I didn't think he was going to because he wasn't taking control of anything. He told me afterwards that he didn't do that because he knew I would've soon clocked the reason why!

I love the free feeling of being outdoors, so Jim decided to propose outside. On 12th December 2012, I suggested we go for a walk through Central Park. It was about midday and a wonderful clear day with no people around. He made the most perfect proposal: he dropped down to one knee and did a little speech, which is just between me and him but safe to say, it was very emotional and I cried a lot, but I said yes straightaway! We then went to one of the big department stores and had a drink and rang our families to tell them the news, but everyone knew! He had asked my dad and there was not one person I told who didn't know before me – naughty Jim! He told me he had had the ring in his pocket for three days, so I didn't stumble across it in the hotel room, and when we went to the Rockefeller Center earlier on our trip Jim kept buzzing when he went through the metal detector but managed to hide it – and the security guard just gave him a wink.

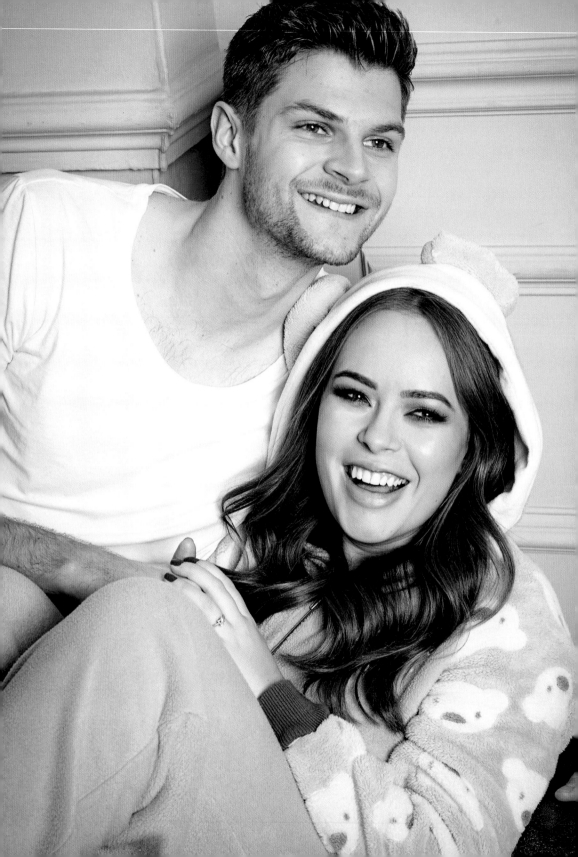

We're planning on getting married later this year. I can't wait to choose my dress but I haven't been shopping yet because I've been so busy with work. I plan to take Mum, Tasha, Judy, Sam and Nic – it's going to be busy in the changing room! I'm so excited about choosing it and am thinking about making some bookings at wedding dress shops. I want to go for something unique and different, not your classic wedding dress. I might totally change my mind but, at the moment, that's the plan.

I've always had a thing about getting married outside, so we're really hoping for good weather. We're planning a really private, intimate ceremony with just sixty of our closest family and friends and I won't be doing a video of it, but I plan to give my viewers a sneak peek at some of the aspects of the day. I'm so excited to be marrying my soulmate and favourite person in the world.

MY TOP 10
DATE IDEAS

1 | ICE-SKATING/ROLLER-BLADING

I love physical dates where you can bond over how good or bad you are at the activity. If you are rubbish, it doesn't matter because you can cling onto your date and laugh about it together.

2 | CINEMA/THEATRE

This is a good option if you are nervous about making conversation because watching a film or seeing a show gives you something to talk about afterwards. If you don't know each other very well then maybe save it for the second or third date, because the last thing you want to be doing if you've never met the person properly is to be sitting in a dark room not talking to each other for two hours! My favourite film is Quentin Tarantino's *True Romance*; it's so cool.

3 | DINNER

Dinner is always at the top of my list when it comes to dates. I love trying out new places to eat, but do be careful what you choose to eat. In the vlog where I announced this book, Jim and I were cooking spaghetti bolognese – be warned that this is not a good choice for first date food because it makes such a mess and ends up down your chin!

4 BIKE RIDE AND PICNIC IN THE PARK

This is the perfect summer date because picnics allow for a natural and relaxed vibe. There's no set routine, so if it's going well, you can watch the world go by and end up chatting for hours.

5 FEEDING CUTE ANIMALS AT A FARM

There are, of course, the big zoos but for an inexpensive and relaxed day out, check out the local (city) farm. Many farms rely on visitors to stay open and there is often an opportunity to feed the goats and lambs.

6 ART GALLERIES

I really enjoy looking around art galleries at the different exhibitions and this would make a really relaxed date. London is brilliant for galleries and you can visit so many of them for free. Jim and I enjoy going to the Tate galleries and the Saatchi Gallery.

7 BEACH

The beach has always been a favourite destination of mine. Jim and I go and eat fish and chips and ice creams on Southwold Pier, so if you live near the beach and are meeting someone special, this could be the perfect place to do the same thing.

8 | CLASSES

Whether it's chocolate making, pottery classes or mixing cocktails, interactive classes are a fab way to learn something new, while also spending time getting to know someone. When we were in Thailand we went on a Thai cooking course and made spring rolls and curry paste.

9 | FESTIVE FUN

One of my favourite events is Winter Wonderland in London, where they have an ice rink, circus, rides and a giant observation wheel. We wrap up warm, drink hot chocolate and have a great time. There are lots of festive events like these around the country.

10 | COUNTRY PUB

I love traditional country pubs where you can get a drink and sit in front of a roaring log fire and play board games like Scrabble and Monopoly. Evenings like this can be spontaneous and really fun.

MY TOP 10
RELATIONSHIP TIPS

1 | REALLY TRY TO SEE THE OTHER PERSON'S POINT OF VIEW

It's good to remember that everyone doesn't think the same way as you. Just because you think about something a certain way, doesn't mean your partner will do the same. Every person is very different and I've come to learn that Jim doesn't think in exactly the way I do.

2 | ALWAYS GO ON DATE NIGHTS

When you're busy, it's very easy to not spend enough quality time with your partner. Date nights are so important, so block out a date in your diary and make sure you spend some quality time alone together. You don't need to go out and do anything particularly special – although that is great, too! – sometimes just sitting and chatting over a meal can be a good way of re-connecting with your partner.

3 | DON'T LET YOUR LAPTOP AND PHONE COME BETWEEN YOU

If you are spending quality time with your other half, make sure you have a laptop or phone amnesty. Jim and I always make sure we put our phones away if we are going out for a nice dinner. It's a good idea to have some no-phone zones and make sure one of these is the bedroom.

4 | MAKE SMALL GESTURES

Treating each other by buying little gifts and cards can make them feel so special and appreciated. Jim knows that I hate it when a big event is over because I love having something to look forward to, and when I got back home from my lash launch at the end of last October he had put a dark-green velvet Harrods stocking on the end of my bed with some chocolate money in it. He had put a card there too, saying, 'Christmas is coming, get excited!'

5 | TRY TO BE KIND TO EACH OTHER

I think lots of couples take out their stresses and frustrations on each other and their default mode is to be like that. I think it's really important to always try and be kind to each other. Try and be there for each other and treat each other well.

6 | NEVER GO TO BED ON AN ARGUMENT

This old-school bit of advice is a really good one, I think, because going to bed when you are angry and tired is a really bad combination. Jim and I did this recently after a silly argument and I ended up lying in bed for ages feeling annoyed with him.

7 | ALWAYS COMMUNICATE

If you are worried about the relationship for any reason, make sure you talk it through with your partner, so they can reassure you. Honest and open communication also ensures there are no misunderstandings between you.

8 | ALWAYS HAVE TIME APART

When I first got together with Jim, I spent less time with my girlfriends, but I think it is so important to have separate interests and friends. Jim and I always spend time doing different things. I regularly have girls' nights with either Kate, Maddie, Vanessa and Emma, or Niomi and Zoe, and I think this is a really good thing for my relationship.

9 | KEEP IT LIGHT-HEARTED

Try to enjoy your time together and not be too serious all the time. Even if Jim is in the shower and I am brushing my teeth getting ready to go, we try to make some fun out of this time and sing silly songs.

10 | SHARE CHORES

If you live together, always try to pitch in and help. There is always some stuff that you don't like doing and some stuff that you don't mind doing – and it is just a case of finding out what those things are. Jim likes doing the washing because he likes organising it and I do the dishwasher a lot more than him. But we do still manage to argue about mess around the house sometimes! He gets annoyed if I leave the toothpaste tube with toothpaste popping out of the top and I get frustrated with him for leaving random things like his hair gel on the dining table.

MY TOP 10
TIPS ON DRESSING FOR A FIRST DATE

1 | **MAKE A PLAN**
Always try to find out what you are going to do so you can plan an outfit and make sure you have tried on what you are planning to wear beforehand. If you can't decide, get a friend to take photos.

2 | **BE COMFORTABLE**
If you are going on a cinema date, then I would wear leggings and Converse so that I was comfortable and then add something to give my outfit an edge, like a blazer or a statement necklace. If you're comfortable you will be able to relax and be yourself.

3 | **DON'T GO TOO HIGH**
If you are going for dinner, don't wear sky-high heels because there is nothing worse than standing up to go to the loo and thinking you might topple over!

4 | **KEEP THE MYSTERY**
Less is always more. I don't ever wear a short skirt and low-cut top and keeping one or the other area covered adds to your air of mystery.

5 | **BE YOURSELF**
Don't dress for what you think your date will like but dress for yourself. For example, if they're a huge rock fan, don't turn up in a rock T-shirt and studded

belt if you're a girly girl. If the relationship goes somewhere, then they're going to get to know you for who you are anyway. Play up your own unique style and be yourself!

6 | KEEP YOUR MAKE-UP EASY
Don't do a make-up look that needs constant touching-up. By all means, give yourself smoky eyes because that's easy, but make sure you have waterproof mascara on. I would always choose lip gloss over lipstick.

7 | DON'T OVERDO YOUR HAIR
For a first date you want to look like you've made a big effort but don't go too OTT with a complicated up-do.

8 | FEEL AMAZING
No matter what you are wearing, you should feel amazing. If you do, your date will pick up on it and think you are pretty great, too!

9 | DON'T GO NEW
Even if you really want the date to go well, it's not necessary to go out and buy a whole new wardrobe. Wear an existing favourite outfit.

10 | THINK OF THE SMALL DETAILS
For me, things like having my nails painted, wearing a cool necklace and spending a few minutes longer on my make-up, makes me feel great and I think it's the small things that can give you a pre-date boost.

NOTES

List your favourite romantic films...

♡

NOTES

List date-night ideas you want to try...

♡

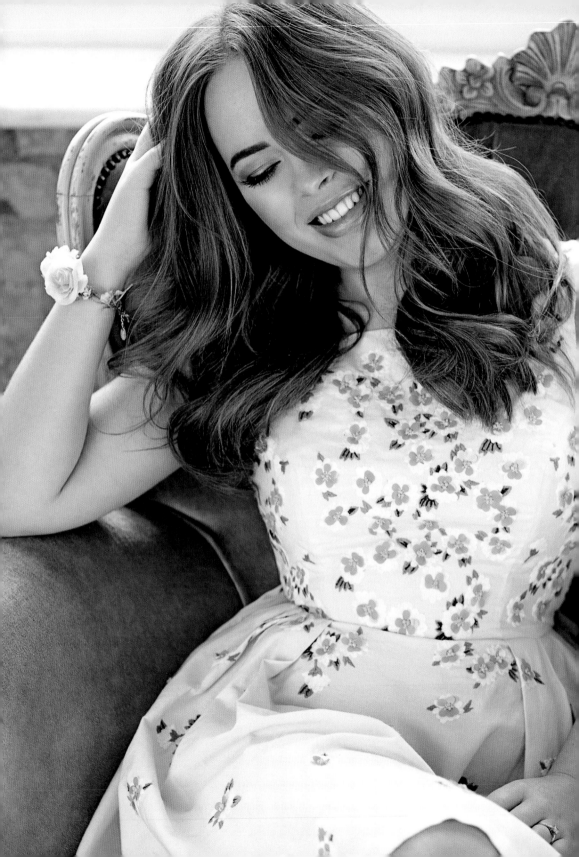

LIFE

FRIENDSHIPS

Growing up, I would see my best friends every day after school until I was eighteen. If you're at school and reading this, make the most of those times because these are often the friends who will be your lifelong allies. After school, we all took different paths and most of my friends went off to university: Maddie went to Manchester, Emma and Kate came down to London, and I was still working and living in Norwich. I still made a big effort to keep in touch with them and I think this is so important; we would speak on the phone and see each other as much as possible. I remember staying in Kate's single bed with her at her university halls!

I was also lucky enough to have a best friend in my sister. Like most siblings, we had our moments in our teenage years when we didn't get on and hated the sight of each other, but this always only ever lasted a few hours and we are closer than ever. If you have a sibling, treasure them always because they will be your friends for life.

Aside from my friends from home, I have formed some really good friendships with other YouTubers. When my video work really started taking off, I started to be invited to different conventions all around the world, like VidCon, which is held annually in LA, and Playlist Live, an annual YouTube gathering in Florida. The purpose of these events is to bring together creators, viewers and industry representatives and we would always be put up in the same hotel. It feels a bit like a school trip, where you all spend loads of time together. A lot of YouTubers in the UK are looked after by my management team, so in the early days we would often bump into each other at different meetings or see one another around the Gleam office in Shoreditch.

My friendship with Zoe started back in 2012. Alfie and Jim were chatting on Twitter and they decided that it would be fun to film a video together where Alfie lived with his mum and dad in Brighton. I went along with Jim and we stayed at a hotel called Drake's because at this point we didn't know Alfie well enough to stay with him. It felt a bit like we were on holiday because I hadn't been to Brighton before. We explored The Lanes and I loved it because everywhere was so cutesy and pretty. It also reminded me a bit of Harry Potter's Knockturn Alley, which made me like it even more!

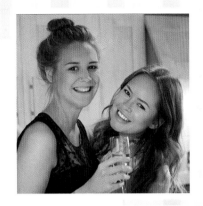

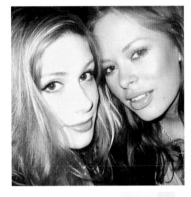

We found Alfie's mum's house and Zoe was there as she was friends with Alfie at the time and she was visiting him, too. Zoe and I had met in London for tea and cake about a month before and we had just really hit it off and after a couple of hours chatting it was as if I'd known her all my life. She's the kind of girl I knew I would have been best friends with if we had been at school together. So while the boys filmed their videos we went into another room and chatted away. After they had finished filming their video, we all decided to record some more videos all together and ended up spending the whole evening messing

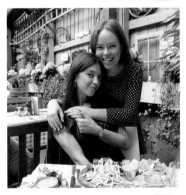

around on camera with them and ordering Domino's. As a foursome, we had loads in common and when Jim and I eventually got back to our hotel late that night, we knew we had made some brilliant friends. Not long afterwards, we invited them to come and stay with us at our home in Norwich and we had such a fun time. We had a barbecue in the garden, showed them around the city centre and filmed a load of videos together. None of our little group of YouTube friends lives near each other, so after our initial meetings, we would always invite each other to come and stay for weekends and so got to know each other really quickly. It was great getting to know Alfie and Zoe because most of my friends at the time were single and it was good to spend time with another couple. From then on, we kept in touch loads through Skype and are always planning the next time we're going to see each other.

During one trip to Zoe's parents' house near Bath, I met her younger brother Joe and we also got on really well. Joe had trained to be a roof thatcher but had started making YouTube videos. Alfie and another American YouTuber Tyler Oakley were also staying. Again, we just had such a great time making videos together and went on walks, ate ice cream and explored the local area. Now, the relationship I have with Joe is a bit of a brother–sister one. He lives in London and I like to look out for him and cook him dinner, even if 'dinner' is just peanut butter on toast!

Another couple in our little close group of YouTube friends are Marcus and Niomi. Marcus has been doing videos on YouTube for years and we would always hang out in groups. His girlfriend Niomi then started posting

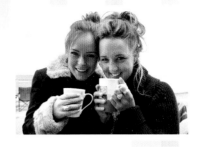

her own videos and spending more time with us. One day Marcus and I wanted to film together so they came to stay with us in Norwich. Niomi and I were domestic goddesses and had some really funny times in the kitchen. She and Marcus love healthy food so we decided to make my healthy chocolate brownies. When all the chocolate had melted in the pot, just as I was checking the recipe on my blog, I told her to put everything else in.

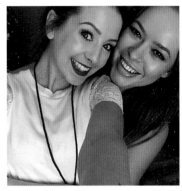

As I turned around, I was saying, 'apart from the eggs!' but obviously she had already put the eggs into this boiling mixture and they all scrambled, so we renamed them scrambled egg brownies! Meanwhile, the boys spent the entire time on their PlayStations and in the evening we would all sit around and watch TV together. At the time, one of Jim and my favourite TV shows was *The Vampire Diaries* and we really got them into it. They are still obsessed with it now. Last year Zoe and Alfie, Marcus and Niomi and Jim and I went on holiday together to Santorini and had such a relaxing time lounging around reading, sunbathing and catching up – there is never any drama and we always just have so much fun.

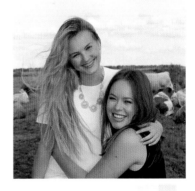

I also have some other special friendships with YouTubers around the world, such as Connor Franta, Tyler Oakley, Troye Sivan,

Joey Graceffa and Ingrid Nilsen, and we all keep in touch via Skype and text. I've been to stay with Ingrid in LA and I am planning a trip to see Troye in Australia later this year. At any possible opportunity when they are over in the UK or we are planning work trips abroad, we always make time to see one another.

Of course there are other YouTube stars who I work and really get on with but it would be impossible to mention everyone – and I would hate to miss anyone out! The great thing about my friendship with other YouTubers is that we understand each other and our lives, the highs and lows of having videos on the Internet and the craziness of it all.

One of my rules about friendship is never to gossip. When you're at school, there is so much gossip going around and people trying to be the first to announce news and it's so easy to get drawn in. I think it's so important to not talk about people when they're not there and to speak out against it. It may take guts, but questioning gossip is a really good thing.

I really cherish all my friendships and try to see my best friends as much as I can. Even when it comes to those people who I don't see as much as I'd like, I always keep in touch via text, and when we do see each other face-to-face, it's always as if no time has passed at all. I try not to take anyone for granted. I recently read an article that said friends are essential for our lives, contribute to our physical, emotional and mental wellbeing and even help us live longer. I love this concept!

NOTES

*List your best friends and what
they mean to you...*

♡

TRAVELLING

As a child, we always had family holidays in the UK and I didn't travel on a plane until I was a teenager. My first big trip abroad was to Thailand and Australia with Jim. We booked our tickets with STA Travel and set ourselves a strict budget, with basic hostels and sleep trains and definitely no luxury food.

I had heard Bangkok was intense, but nothing could have prepared me for what it was really like! It was incredibly humid and the roads were so busy. I just remember Jim and I carrying our massive rucksacks looking for somewhere to stay and weaving our way along the Khao San Road, between all the colourful street food stands, market stalls with people trying to sell us stuff and the sea of people and tourists. The noise was unreal and I must've looked like a rabbit caught in the headlights! We saw so many amazing places like Chiang Mai and Koh Phi Phi, which were both stunning. The trip turned out to be such a life-changing experience and I would definitely recommend backpacking as the best way to see a country and discover hidden gems.

One thing I've learned then and since about travelling is to not always head to the very touristy places that everyone says you should visit. In Thailand, we went to Koh Phangan, where the famous Full Moon Parties are held. I really didn't rate it. I'm not a massive party animal and I found the crowds of people drinking loads a bit overwhelming. The other place that I was expecting to enjoy more than I did was Los Angeles. I know it's the entertainment capital of the world, but I found it so huge. Hollywood also felt a bit strange and not how I imagined.

In the last couple of years, I've been so lucky to be able to travel all over the world because of my work and have been abroad at least three times a year. I have seen so many different places and met some really interesting people.

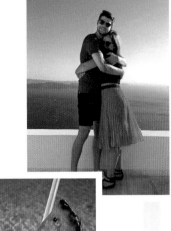

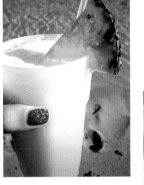

I'm terrible at packing and I used to throw everything into a case but I've had to learn to get better at it, especially as I'm filming myself most days and don't want to wear the same thing loads. My top tip is to plan what you are going to wear each day, rather than think you might have a chance to wear everything and put it in your bag anyway. Niomi gave me this amazing tip recently, which is to lay the outfits out on the bed, complete with shoes and accessories, as you pack and then to photograph them. It means you don't really have to think about what you are going to wear and can just flick through your phone and choose an outfit. Easy! When we were travelling together recently she sent me all her outfits that way, so I could see what she was wearing, and since then, I have done this for every trip I go on.

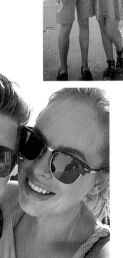

MY TOP 10
FAVOURITE PLACES

1 | SOUTHWOLD
I know I've mentioned this Norfolk town more than once already, but a list of the places I love really wouldn't be complete without it. It holds loads and loads of family memories, but I have also had many great times with my friends here, where we would hang out at my parents' caravan late at night and drink wine and chat. Then we would go onto the beach in the middle of the night and try and scare each other by telling ghost stories!

2 | NORWICH
When I'm in Norwich, I always feel like I know it like the back of my hand and there's something very comforting about that familiarity. I know lots of people in the city and Jim's mum still lives there, so whenever we head back there, we always stay at her house.

3 | LONDON
This is my new home and it's such an exciting place to live. I used to be quite scared of London growing up because it always seemed so big and intimidating. Now I know it better and have found areas that I love like Chelsea, Notting Hill and Primrose Hill. London has such an amazing vibe and feeling of endless possibility about it.

4 | NEW YORK
I first went to New York back in April 2012 with another

YouTuber and friend called Fleur; we met up with Ingrid there and we all stayed at the same hotel. I had wanted to visit the city for ages since my love of *Gossip Girl* and other TV shows, and together we discovered all the best parts of the city, like Central Park, all the shops and restaurants. Even the yellow taxis got me so excited! Jim and I enjoyed it so much that we booked to go back again that same year, when we got engaged. One of my favourite shops is called Henry Bendel's, which is this really glamorous and ornate shop selling jewellery, handbags, fashion accessories and gifts. Recently Jim went to stay in New York and was staying in southern Manhattan, quite a long way from Fifth Avenue where the store is located, but he walked for miles and spent ages walking up and down trying to find it. He bought me this amazing mug with the Henry Bendel's trademark stripes and it makes me so happy when I use it.

5 | PARIS

I first went to Paris on a school trip when I was in the sixth form. I was having quite a hard time generally because I was feeling quite anxious but I felt really happy the whole time I was there on that trip and felt like I turned a bit of a corner; I didn't feel panicky there at all because I was so immersed in the city. I love the art galleries in Paris, like the Rodin Museum, because it is outside, which is pretty cool and, like London and New York, there is so much to see and do. Jim surprised me with a trip there for my twenty-second birthday and we had a magical three days.

6 | MYKONOS, GREECE

Jim and I went on holiday here with Zoe and Alfie in 2013. It was an ordinary holiday and we all took a complete break from vlogging and our hectic schedules for a few days, which felt like bliss. The island is so beautiful and everyone there was so friendly and accommodating. We spent a lot of time just chilling out by the pool, and the hotel that we stayed at, called Bill & Coo, was so tranquil and luxurious. Another big plus was that the island is just a few hours' flight away and is so tiny that our journey to the hotel literally took about five minutes. It was one of our best holidays.

7 | NORTH NORFOLK

We often used to take daytrips to North Norfolk when I was growing up but I have better memories of the area from times spent there with my friends when I was slightly older. I particularly like Holkham because of the stunning forests and beach, where you have to walk for about a mile to get to the sea. There are some lovely sites to see like Holkham Hall, a grand eighteenth-century house, which is surrounded by acres of rolling countryside and wild deer. We took Niomi and Marcus there recently for a day of fresh air, sunshine, yummy food, beach walking and tree climbing. The other place we like in the area is this really vibrant and trendy village called Burnham Market. We always go to a luxury boutique hotel called The Hoste Arms; the food there is delicious.

8 | BABINGTON HOUSE, SOMERSET

I know that everywhere else on this list is a village or town, but I had to mention Babington House. I love open spaces and it turns out the 'house' is actually an incredibly beautiful mansion with eighteen acres of British countryside, tennis courts, a cricket pitch and a walled garden. The rooms are all different and unique and there is a really relaxed and intimate vibe about it. When we stayed there we had this incredible huge room, with massive comfortable sofas, then a winding staircase leading up to a mezzanine bedroom area. The staff were so friendly and the food was delicious and there was free afternoon tea from 3–5 p.m. every day. Jim and I also I did this crazy couples mud treatment thing where we took all our clothes off and covered each other in cleansing mud in our own private steam room! I am planning another trip there and I can't wait!

9 | CANNES

Cannes is super-glamorous and flashy but rather than the plush restaurants and hotels, my favourite thing about it is the sea! The first thing I do after we arrive is jump straight in the sea and swim out as far as I can. I am also a massive fan of fireworks and Jim and I have been for Bastille Day or French National Day, which is on 14th July, for the past couple of years, just for a couple of days. We always go for a lovely dinner and then sit and watch the fireworks from the balcony of our hotel or from the beach. The French really know how to throw a fireworks party!

Another top tip: if you visit, there is this ice cream place called Le Quirly that sells the most yummy ice cream – the Ferrero Rocher flavour is so good!

10 | MANHATTAN BEACH

Last year, after Vidcon, we stayed on in America with our friend Ingrid to catch up and chill out for a few days. One day we headed to Manhattan Beach and really enjoyed it. As I said before, I wasn't crazy about LA, but I could live in Manhattan Beach – it was really quirky with gorgeous cafés, lots of adorable New American-style houses and a beautiful beach.

NOTES

List your top ten things to bring on holiday...

♡

NOTES

List your favourite places in the world...

- -

- -

- -

- -

- -

- -

- -

- -

- -

- -

- -

- -

- -

- -

- -

- -

- -

♡

NOTES

List places you could see yourself living...

♡

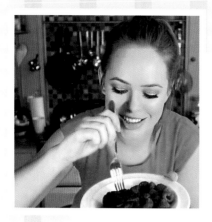
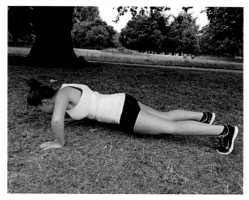

FOOD AND EXERCISE

Having beautiful skin and feeling good about your body all begins with a healthy lifestyle. Basics like eating the right kind of foods, drinking plenty of water and getting enough exercise are the key to looking and feeling good. As I've grown up I've become much more at peace with my body and have found a healthy eating lifestyle that suits me. I always find the best way to tell if I'm in shape is by the way my clothes fit. If you're working out, the figure on the scales is irrelevant because muscle weighs more than fat. I've come to understand that even if I was to exercise and starve myself, I'm never going to have the skinniest thighs or grow really long legs. I've learned to love and respect my body and even if I do have an extra slice of cake, I don't beat myself up about it. Nobody's perfect and you shouldn't have to be. For me, the key to being healthy is finding a happy balance.

EXERCISE

The human body is designed to move and whether you are sitting down at school, doing an office job or, like me, spend hours at a time on your laptop, it is important to try and incorporate exercise into your day. In terms of exercise I work out with my trainer, Russell Bateman, once a week and I also work out with Jim sometimes or do workouts at home. Instead of spending loads of money having Russ train me four times a week (which is how often I try to work out), he will randomly text me and say, 'Got time for a fifteen-minute workout?' Then he'll text me instructions for what to do in my flat! You don't need to be good at sport to exercise – I'm proof of this. I was dreadful at sports at school and was always in tears on Sports Day because I came last in everything, even the egg and spoon race!

The great thing about exercise is that it will trigger feel-good endorphins, which help lift your spirits and give you that feel-good feeling and I always feel better about my body when I've worked up a good sweat. Sometimes it's hard to find time to exercise between school, work or other responsibilities that get in the way. I always try to schedule time in my diary, even if it is just half an hour of yoga before I go out for an evening. The recommended guideline is half an hour of moderate exercise four times a week and whatever you do, try to stick to it so it becomes a habit. As well as not obsessing over the scales, I think it is easy to get preoccupied with the machines at the gym that tell you you have burned off a certain number of calories. And sometimes staring at an empty wall while pounding away on the treadmill can get pretty boring even for the most hard-core gym bunnies, but different exercise regimes work for different people. Whatever you do, just get moving and have fun with it.

MY TOP 10
FUN WAYS TO GET FIT

1 | DO AN EXERCISE VIDEO

This is a really good way of easing yourself into exercise if you are worried about running outside or joining a gym. I went through a phase of doing one of Davina McCall's fitness DVDs every day, and one day when my friends came over and I hadn't done my exercise that day, I made them do it with me. Jim and I have done the *Insanity* DVD together – it was pretty hardcore!

2 | DO CIRCUITS

Make up your own boot camp in the local park and incorporate strength and cardio exercises. Recently Jim and I headed out to the local park and did our own circuit with push-ups, running, sit-ups and jumping jacks and it was really fun. Try to keep your heart rate high by not giving yourself much rest time between circuits for the best results.

3 | JOIN A CLUB

I always love exercising in a group. By joining the local tennis, netball or running club, you will not only get fit but make some new friends as well.

4 | HIT THE SHOPS

Next time you hit the shops, leave the car at home or get off the bus a stop earlier and make sure you carry all your bags to give your arms a good workout.

5 | WALK THE DOG

I always used to walk my dogs when I was younger and could never get out of it, but once I was outside, it felt good being out in the fresh air and I always felt refreshed when I got home. If you don't have a dog, borrow a friend's or hire yourself out as a dog walker for neighbours.

6 | PUT ON YOUR DANCING SHOES

Whether it's making up routines in your own home with friends, heading out to a Zumba class or hitting the dance floor on a night out, dancing can be a brilliant calorie-burner and good fun. This is maybe a bit embarrassing, but sometimes I like to put on one of my favourite albums and Jim and I just dance around the bedroom while we get ready in the morning. It puts me in the best mood and is so uplifting.

7 | MAKE FRIENDS WITH YOUR HOOVER

I'm not a massive fan of cleaning but boring jobs like vacuuming can work your upper body and tone your shoulders and biceps, while ironing and gardening are also good calorie-burners.

8 | CATCH UP ON THE GO

Instead of calling your friends to have a chat, arrange to have a power-walk instead. You'll get some quality time together and bond on the go.

9 | MASTER A NEW SKILL

Have you always wanted to learn to roller skate? Or play tennis? Mastering a new sport is a fab way to get into shape without even realising it. Your brain is so focused on what you are doing that you don't notice the effort you are putting in.

10 | EMBRACE YOUR INNER KID

From flying a kite in the park, to hula-hooping or skipping in the back garden, kids' games don't feel like hard work and have loads of fitness benefits. I always jump around on the trampoline with Oscar and my nephew Isaac when I am home in Norfolk.

NOTES

List new activities you want to try...

♡

EATING RIGHT

I live by the 80/20 rule and I try to follow it as closely as possible. What this means is that eighty per cent of the time, I try to eat fresh and healthy foods and not too much sugar, while the other twenty per cent of the time, I treat myself to cookies, cupcakes and cheesy pasta.

Like every girl, I have some bad weeks where I have far more than my twenty per cent of naughty treats and struggle to get back on track. If that happens I have a real detox, where I eat a ton of superfoods and have lots of green juices and veggies and I'm left feeling refreshed, happy and good about my body. I never obsess over the scales. I am a real foodie and I enjoy trying different restaurants and types of cuisines; often I can find myself eating out a few nights a week but I will try and make healthy choices. I don't think there's any such thing as the perfect diet: it's more a case of finding what works best for your lifestyle. Even small changes can have a big effect on your overall health.

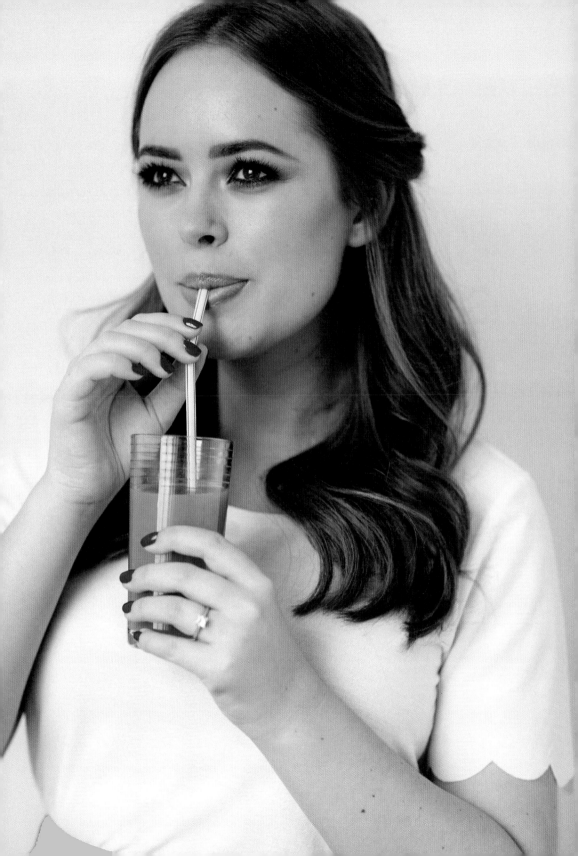

MY TOP 10
HEALTHY EATING TIPS

1 | DON'T SKIP MEALS

Don't eliminate entire meals as it will slow down your metabolism. Your metabolism is like a muscle – use it or you will lose it! When you skip meals and go many hours without eating, your metabolism slows down, so when you do finally eat something, your metabolism can't break down the food so quickly and as a result, the food is stored as fat. Also, skipping meals encourages you to overeat when you do decide to have a meal. Recently I was at Zoe's house and we didn't eat breakfast until 11.30 a.m. and then we worked all day filming videos until about 10 p.m. Then we went to Wagamama's and ate far more than we would have done if we had eaten a normal breakfast and lunch. If I skip a meal, I find myself eating anything in sight!

2 | MAKE HEALTHY SWAPS

Try making small changes to your diet – swap your full-fat ice-cream for frozen yogurt or make your own home-made ice cream with bananas and berries. Even something as simple as picking wholemeal bread rather than white bread will have a positive impact on your health.

3 | MAKE GRADUAL CHANGES

It can be quite daunting when it comes to changing your diet. Make gradual changes, even if you start with one meal at a time. So if you have a diet full of junk food and normally start the day with a large fry-up, try having unsweetened granola and fruit and milk, or poached eggs on wholemeal toast instead and you'll see such a big change. Don't feel under pressure to change everything immediately.

4 | DON'T SKIMP ON SLEEP
Make sure you get at least six to eight hours' sleep a night. Without it the appetite hormone increases, which will make you crave sugary and starchy foods.

5 | EAT SLOWLY
So many of us, me included, are guilty of eating in a rush. Try to eat your food slowly and be mindful of every mouthful. In this way, it is much easier to tell when we have eaten enough and are full.

6 | DON'T DEPRIVE YOURSELF
If you completely deprive yourself of something you really like to eat, you will only crave it more. I try to have everything in moderation and most of the time stick to Sunday as my cheat day, when I am allowed to eat something I have been craving.

7 | PLAN YOUR MEALS
To avoid going for the quick fixes, plan your meals beforehand. Make a shopping list and buy all the ingredients for a week's worth of meals in one go to ensure you have all you need for making your meals.

8 | STAY WELL HYDRATED

The best hydration comes from plain water, soups and watery foods, such as fruit and vegetables. When I am working I always try to keep a large glass of water by my side. If I want a change, I'll add some elderflower cordial.

9 | AIM TO EAT UNPROCESSED FOODS

The best foods for your body are clean, unprocessed foods like fruit and vegetables, lean meat and oily fish. You'll notice if you pick up a chocolate bar, it has about twenty ingredients, whereas an avocado is just one.

10 | HAVE HEALTHY SNACKS

If you get peckish mid-afternoon, a healthy snack can boost your energy levels and stabilise your blood sugar. Always have healthy snacks, like nuts and seeds or a yogurt, to hand so you don't reach for the biscuits. When I'm going to loads of shows at London Fashion Week and it's manically busy, I always take a bag of unsalted almonds with me in my bag and munch away like a squirrel between shows.

NOTES

List some healthy foods that you want to introduce into your diet...

♡

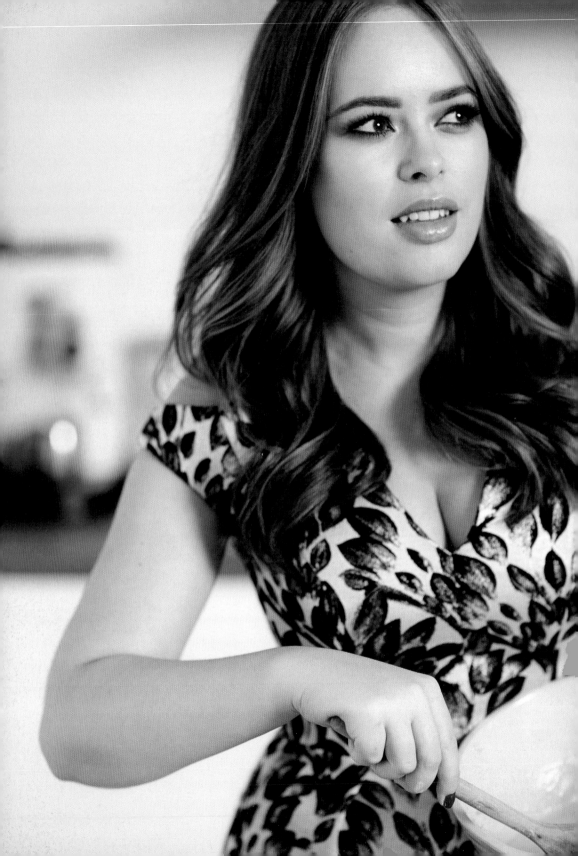

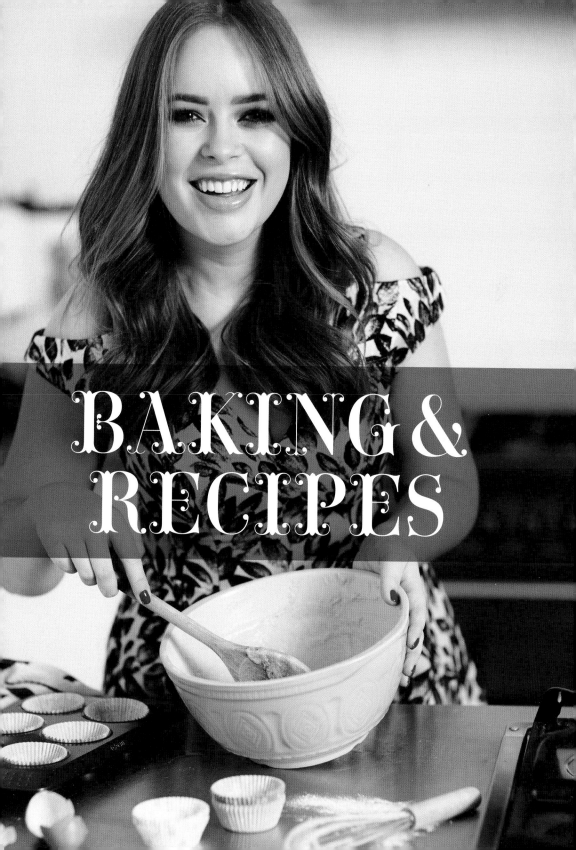

BAKING & RECIPES

Baking was such a big part of my childhood. Some of my earliest and best memories are standing on a chair (so I could reach the kitchen counter) and baking with my mum. We used to make simple recipes like lemon tray bake, fairy cakes and butterfly cakes and I always got to lick the spoon afterwards – the best bit!

When I decided to start doing baking videos on my channel, I wasn't sure whether my viewers would enjoy them. However, my first one got such a good reaction that I started doing some more; often when I do meet-ups, I ask my fans what they love most about my videos and loads of them say baking! I get so excited when I am sent pictures of people making my creations and sometimes I'll post a baking video and for weeks afterwards, viewers will be sending me their cute photos. Sometimes I find it hard to find time to bake and create new recipes but it makes me so happy and calm. Here are some of my favourite recipes for you to enjoy.

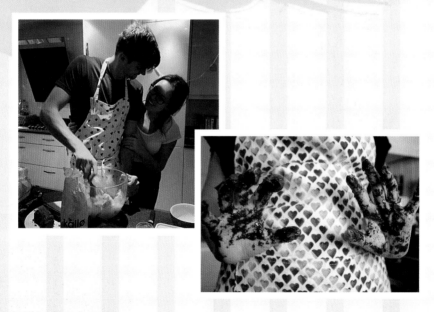

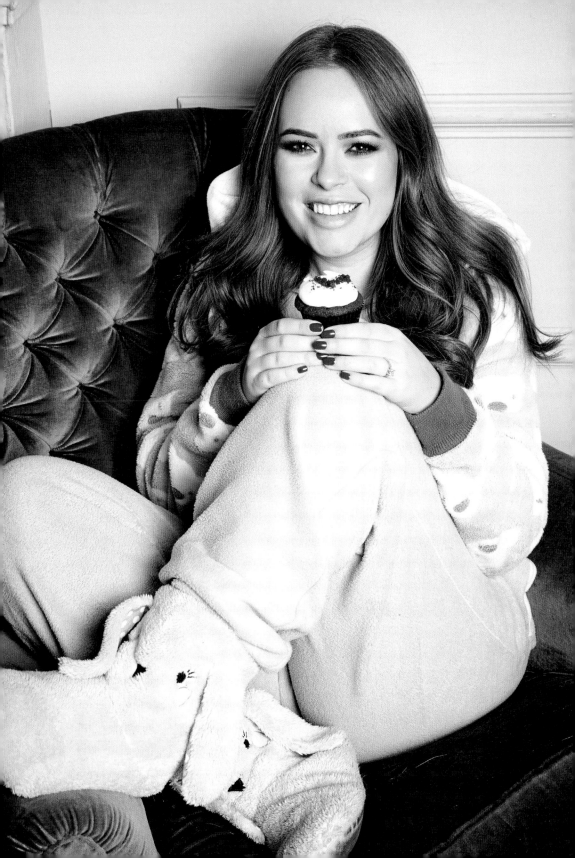

AMAZING CHOCOLATE BROWNIES

The best part about these brownies is they contain much healthier ingredients than traditional brownies. They are still high in calories, so definitely a treat, but they are dairy-free (depending on what type of chocolate you use), gluten-free and made using healthy fats. People get scared of coconut oil as it's high in saturated fat, but I have spoken to Jim's brother John, who knows everything there is to know about food, and he said it's a special type of saturated fat that is actually good for you! My trainer even tries to get me to eat a spoonful of coconut oil before a workout sometimes, but I find it too gross and oily on its own. Avocado is another type of healthy fat and I use it in this recipe to give a creamy texture – you don't taste it, don't worry. The coconut sugar works like regular sugar apart from it being unrefined and so it doesn't spike your blood sugar levels like regular sugar. I am no nutritionist, but these are just some helpful healthy facts I have learned.

**To make nine brownies
you will need:**
½ cup coconut oil
300g dark chocolate
2 cups coconut sugar
1 cup ground almonds
1 teaspoon baking powder
1 mashed avocado
1 capful vanilla extract
Pinch of salt
3 eggs

Pre-heat your oven to 180°C. Then put a large saucepan over a low heat and pop in your coconut oil and chocolate. Once all the chocolate has melted, turn off the heat and add in your coconut sugar, ground almonds, baking powder, avocado (make sure this is really well mashed and stirred in), vanilla extract, salt and eggs. I like to have already beaten the three eggs together in a cup before pouring them in.

Pour your mixture into a tin and pop in the oven for 26 minutes! When you take it out, it should look cooked on top but will still be squishy in the middle. Leave it to cool for 20 minutes then serve with whatever you like. My top serving recommendation is frozen yoghurt and berries.

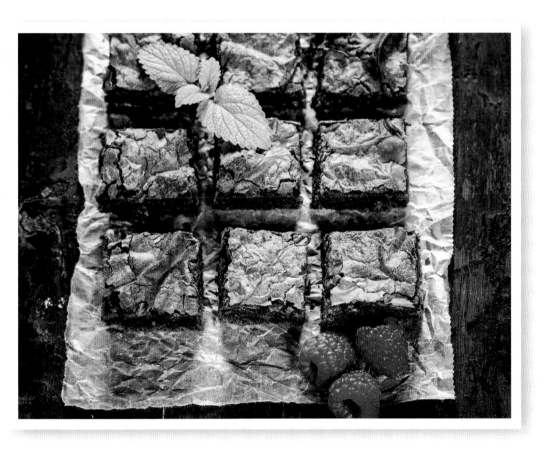

LEMON DRIZZLE LOAF

I used to make this with my mum when I was little because it is one of my dad's favourites so always had a great reception. It's perfect for all year round and is a lovely mix of being moist and crunchy at the same time. Yum!

For the cake:
3 eggs
170g self-raising flour
170g caster sugar
170g butter
1 teaspoon baking powder
Zest of 2 lemons

For the icing:
150g icing sugar
Juice of 2 lemons

Pre-heat your oven to 180°C. Mix the eggs, flour, sugar, butter, baking powder and the zest of two lemons into a big mixing bowl. Line your baking tin with a bit of butter or use a non-stick baking tin and pour mixture in. Bake for 35–45 minutes – the cooking time depends on the size of the tin and your oven. To check your cake is ready, slide a knife into the centre and if it comes out clean, it is ready to come out of the oven.

Mix together the icing sugar and juice of the lemons to make the drizzle. Stir it together – it should be quite a watery consistency. While your cake is still hot, poke it all over with a skewer or sharp knife, and then pour over the drizzle so it can soak in. If I'm having friends over for afternoon tea or want the cake to look extra pretty, I like to dress it with flowers or fruit.

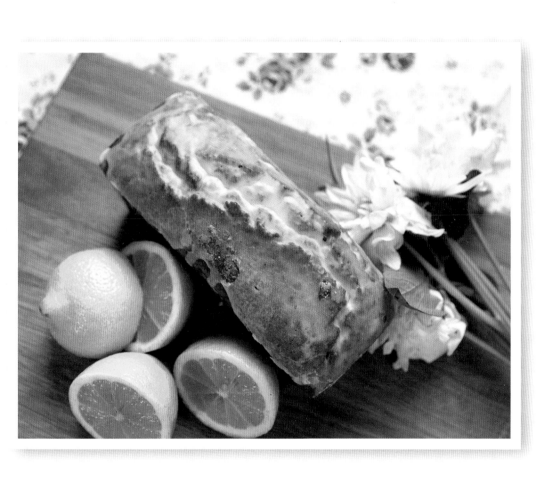

TRIPLE CHOCOLATE COOKIES

Chocolate-based baking is my favourite and I originally baked these cookies on my YouTube channel because I was inspired by something similar I had seen, so I decided to create my own recipe. Here's how you can made a batch of this gooey, chocolatey naughtiness!

To make ten cookies you will need:
200g butter
300g caster sugar
1 large egg
275g self-raising flour
75g cocoa powder
A little dash of milk (optional)
A large bar each of white, milk and dark chocolate
3 Daim bars

Pre-heat your oven to 200°C. Then whizz together your butter and sugar until it's a smooth consistency. Crack in the egg and then put in your dry ingredients and blend it together. If your mixture looks too dry, add some milk.

Now for the chocolate… break it all up and throw into your mixture. Very importantly, don't forget the Daim bars! They give the cookies an incredible and unexpected toffee crunch. Once you've mixed the chocolate in, line two trays with baking paper or foil and then prepare to get messy! Use your hands to separate the mixture into ten blobs.

Now pop your chocolatey blobs in the oven for 11 minutes – I have found this to be the perfect baking time. When you take them out they will not look cooked; it is vital you know this, as it will be very tempting to leave them in for longer and then they'll be hard and overcooked once they are cool. Just take your cookies out after 11 minutes and leave them to cool for about 30 minutes. Use this time to put on one of your favourite soundtracks and dance round the kitchen – Jim and I often sing along to *Drake*. I don't know why, but this album is often our baking soundtrack!

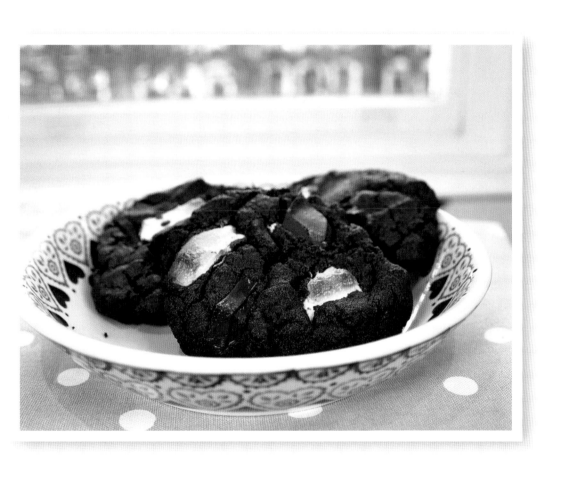

MILK AND WHITE CHOCOLATE COOKIES

These feel like a real treat and everyone needs a treat in their lives! They have a traditional cookie dough base with milk and white chocolate blended in and similar to my chocolate cookies on the previous page. I always make these for Jim and I when we are having a night in, watching Modern Family *or* Vampire Diaries *and we want a sweet treat to go with our tea.*

To make ten cookies you will need:
200g butter
300g caster sugar
1 large egg
325g self-raising flour
A dash of milk (optional)
200g white chocolate (my favourite is Milky Bar but you can use any white chocolate you like)
200g milk chocolate (again, my favourite is Cadbury but use any brand)

Pre-heat your oven to 200°C and then start off by whisking the butter and sugar together until it's pale and creamy. Make sure your butter is at room temperature so it blends easily. Crack in the egg and mix it through. Gradually add the flour by popping in a bit at a time, until it is all mixed in.

The mixture should then come together and look like dough. If it looks too dry, add a dash of milk until it's the right consistency. If the mixture feels too sticky, just add a touch more flour.

With clean hands, break up the chocolate into big and small chunks and add to the mixture. Grab the dough from underneath and spread the chunks through thoroughly. Shape the mixture into ten balls using your hands and put them on a baking tray covered in greaseproof paper.

Bake these for 10–12 minutes but no longer! They will look like they need longer, but don't do it! Leave them on the baking tray or a cooling rack to cool for 25 minutes. They should be gooey on the inside and hard on the outside – so, so good!

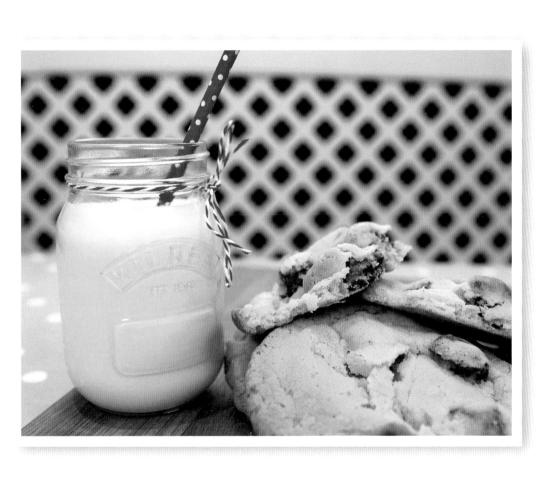

HEALTHY WINTER SOUP

As soon as the clocks go back in the autumn and it starts to get cold and chilly, this is one of the recipes I always turn to because it is so comforting and warm. I start by getting out my fleecy PJs and autumn/winter candles and then cook a homemade soup to warm me up. Homemade soup is great because you can control exactly what you're putting into it. So many ready-made soups that you buy in the supermarket are full of additives and salt. As part of my aim to be healthy eighty per cent of the time, this soup is the perfect thing to cook since as the weather gets colder we tend to start to crave lots of stodgy carbohydrate-based foods like bread, mashed potato and pasta. Because I make this soup quite thick, it ticks the box for me of being that stodgy, warm food but at the same time it is really healthy and tastes great.

You will need:
2 onions
Garlic (put in however
    much you like;
    I did 3 cloves)
A few stalks of celery
Half a head of broccoli
2 leeks
1 large sweet potato
1 carrot
150g red lentils
1 tablespoon olive oil
1 litre chicken stock
Salt and pepper

This is really easy! Just chop up all your veggies and chuck them in the pot. Also pop in the lentils – they are a great source of protein, fibre and loads of vitamins and minerals and they will also help to thicken the soup. Add a bit more oil and then let everything cook for about three minutes.

Now, add a litre of stock – I used chicken stock, but if you are vegetarian you can use veggie stock. Also, if you want to make your soup a bit thinner, just add more stock.

Add salt and pepper and bring it to the boil. Then just let the soup simmer for about 25 minutes or until the sweet potato is soft and the lentils are cooked.

Then use a handheld blender or what I call a 'whizzer' to blend the cooked ingredients and make them into soup! I like my soup quite thick and a bit chunky so I am careful not to whizz mine too much so it still has chunks of veggies in it.

Light one of your favourite wintery candles and cosy up with a bowl of the soup!

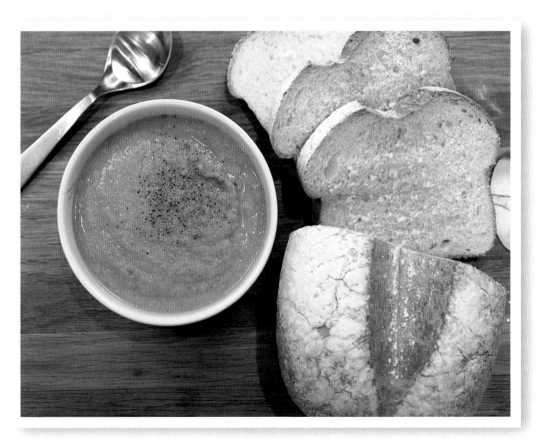

ROASTED SQUASH, LENTIL AND GOAT'S CHEESE SALAD

Jim's mum makes this for us and it's a salad that's great for all year round. It's really filling and satisfying so I never feel hungry afterwards. Again, this is another great option for the eighty per cent of the time that I am trying to be good and the individual ingredients are really nutritious.

You will *need*:
A large butternut squash
Olive oil
Salt and pepper
100g goat's cheese
250g pack of ready-to-eat puy lentils
A handful of cherry tomatoes, chopped
70g spinach
Balsamic vinegar

Pre-heat the oven to 200°C. Line a large baking sheet with baking parchment. Chop up the squash into small chunks and cover with two tablespoons of olive oil and salt and pepper (use as much or as little as you like). Cook for 30–40 minutes.

Break up the goat's cheese into bite-size pieces. Tip the roasted squash into a salad bowl and stir in the lentils, chopped cherry tomatoes, spinach and goat's cheese. Dress with balsamic vinegar and a bit more olive oil to taste. Serve with a smile!

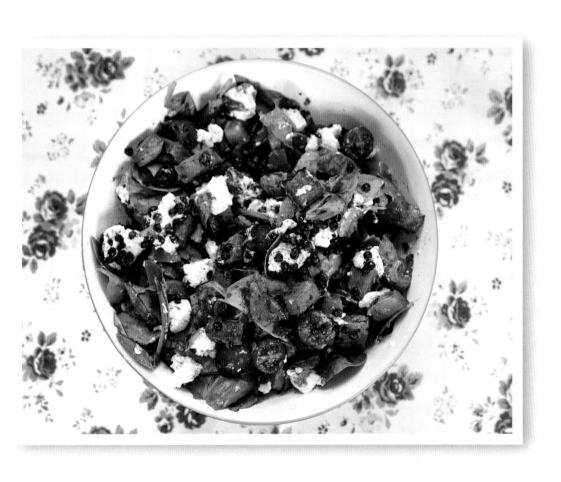

SUNDAY CAKE

This is a cake that Mum made for us every Sunday growing up and for birthdays and special occasions. She would always make it in the morning ready for our family who would come over to our house every Sunday, and she'd mix up the decorations for extra fun.

You will need:
For the cake:
170g butter
170g caster sugar
3 eggs
30g cocoa powder
140g self-raising flour
1½ teaspoons baking
    powder

For the inside icing:
60g butter
110g icing sugar
Cocoa powder to taste

For the topping:
A 200g bar of chocolate
    to melt, and chocolates
    like Smarties, white
    chocolate buttons or
    Maltesers to decorate

Pre-heat the oven to 180°C. Line two baking tins with baking parchment. Cream the butter and sugar together. Then add the eggs, sifted cocoa, flour and baking powder and mix well. Divide the mixture into two baking tins and pop into the oven for 18–20 minutes or until an inserted skewer comes out clean.

For the icing, whisk the butter, icing sugar and cocoa powder together, and for the topping, melt the chocolate in a bowl over simmering water.

When the cake is cool, sandwich the two sides together with the icing and pour the melted chocolate over the top. Decorate with whatever you have in your cupboard – I always love white chocolate buttons on mine.

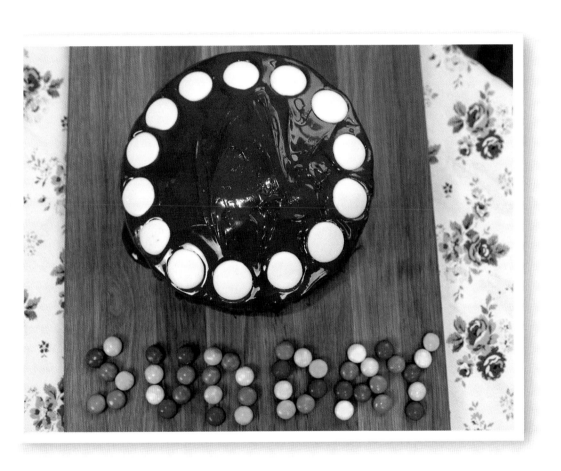

NANNY'S APPLE PIE

When I was little, Nanny always used to cook apple pie for after Sunday lunch every week or if we had lunch at our house, she would always bring one. Out of the whole family I was the most crazy about this pie and always looked forward to it. Now she is older, she doesn't cook as much as she used to and, up until recently, I hadn't had her apple pie for years. Then, a few months ago, when I was in Norfolk, I knew I needed to see her, so Jim and I went over to her house and when we arrived, she pulled an apple pie out of the oven. I thought it was such a sweet gesture and, of course, it tasted amazing! Just the taste of it reminds me of childhood.

You will need:
340g self-raising flour
110g vegetable fat
60g butter
6 tablespoons cold water
5 cooking apples
2 tablespoons
    granulated sugar
1 tablespoon cold water
1 egg

Pre-heat your oven to 200°C. Mix the flour, fat and butter with your fingertips until it turns into a breadcrumb-like consistency. Then add the six tablespoons of water and make into a ball of pastry; wrap in tin foil and put in the fridge for 30 minutes.

Take the apples and peel and chop them. As Nanny chops them, she drops the pieces into a pan of cold water with a pinch of salt to stop them browning. Then rinse the apples and put them in a different pan over a high heat with a tablespoon of water. Add the sugar and simmer for about 10 minutes until soft.

Cool the apple by putting the pan in cold water, then take your pastry from the fridge. Cut the pastry into two pieces, one slightly bigger than the other.

Grease a 10-inch pie dish and roll the larger half of the pastry out. Put it into the bottom of the dish, tuck in the edges and cut any excess pastry away with a blunt knife. Place the apples in the centre of the pie. Take the egg and whisk it, then use the egg mix to moisten the edge of the pastry, before rolling out the other half of pastry and laying it on top. Pierce a hole in the centre to let out the air. Then brush egg over the entire pie and if you want, add a pretty design around the edge of the pie with the leftover pastry – Nanny always does apple leaves.

Bake for 20 minutes and then turn the oven down to 170°C for the last 10 minutes until the pie is golden brown. You can serve it with whatever you fancy, Nanny always serves her pie with custard – heaven!

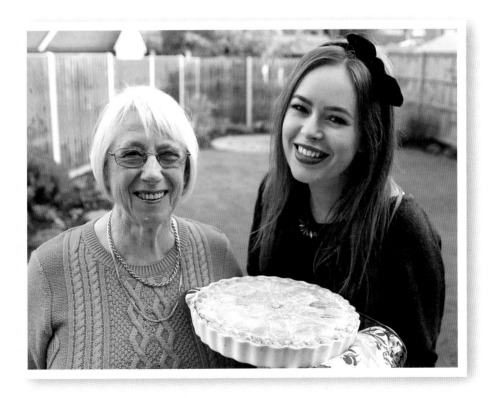

VANILLA STAR-SPRINKLED CUPCAKES

These cupcakes are one of the first cakes I made with my mum when I was small. It was always the perfect snack when I got back from school and I would have it with a glass of squash, but now I'm more partial to having a cup of tea with my cupcake!

To make twelve cupcakes you will need:
For the cupcakes
50g butter
180g caster sugar
160g plain flour
2 teaspoons baking
   powder
160ml milk
1 egg
A few drops of vanilla
   extract (depending on
   how strong you like
   the vanilla flavour)

For the icing:
500g icing sugar
250g butter
½ teaspoon vanilla
   extract

For the decoration:
white and dark chocolate
   stars, edible glitter or
   anything else you like

Pre-heat the oven to 180°C. Cream the butter and sugar together. Then fold in the flour and baking powder and slowly add the milk. Crack in the egg, followed by the vanilla extract and continue beating the mixture throughout.

Spoon the mixture into the twelve cupcake cases and bake for 20 minutes. The baking time varies but they should be golden brown and if you touch them, they should bounce back. Leave them to cool on a wire rack.

Then, for the icing, just mix all the ingredients together and either spoon on top or if you are feeling fancy, use a piping bag to pipe the icing on for a more professional-looking finish. Decorate however you like – my favourites are white and dark chocolate stars and I also have a small obsession with edible glitter, which looks divine!

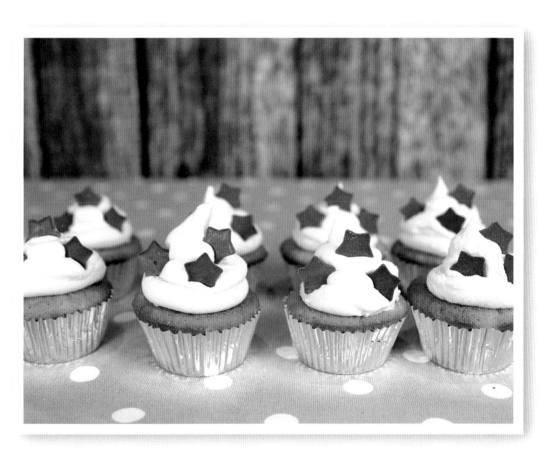

OVERNIGHT OATS BREAKFAST SUNDAE

This reminds me of being in Sydney when I stayed with my cousin Vanessa and her husband Russ because they have these gorgeous breakfast bars on the beach. There was one that we loved just off Bondi Beach where overnight oats, where you soak oats in apple juice, always featured on the menu. It is so fresh, tasty and healthy – the perfect to way to start your day! It's also great if you are short of time in the morning because you can eat it on the go on the bus or at your desk at work.

You will need:
1 large Bramley apple
85g oats
1 cup of almond milk
Two tablespoons honey
One teaspoon cinnamon
2 large handfuls of
    blackberries

Peel the apple and chop into chunks. Put the pieces into a saucepan with a dash of water and simmer until they become soft. This normally takes about 8–10 minutes. If the apples are still lumpy after that time, mash them with a fork and drain off any excess water.

Mix the oats, almond milk, one tablespoon of honey and the cinnamon together and then stir in the apple mixture.

Now move onto the blackberry compôte. Blend the blackberries and one tablespoon of honey in a blender. Take your sundae glass and layer the two mixtures one after the other. I like to mix: oats, compôte, oats then compôte dressed with a single blackberry on top but you can do any combination you choose. Pop the glass in the fridge for at least six hours. This is the perfect recipe to make before bedtime and then you can roll out of bed the next morning and grab your oats before you head out.

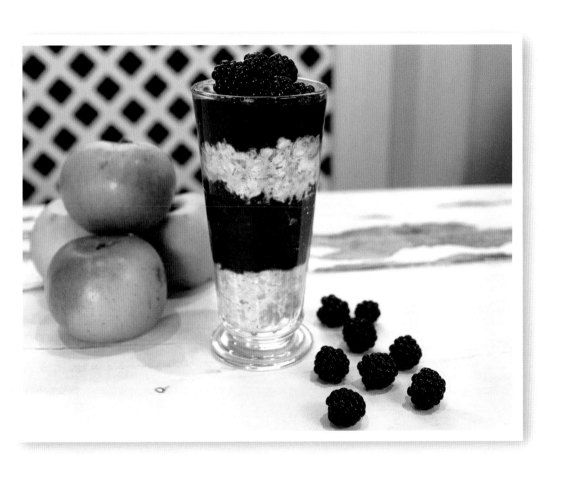

SMARTIES FLAPJACKS

Flapjacks are something I've always made growing up and they remind me of my piano teacher, Mrs Fisher. Before my lessons, she had always been baking and sometimes I would arrive an hour before my piano lesson to eat her flapjacks and play with the other children who were there. These include my own unique chocolatey addition!

For nine flapjacks you will need:
125g butter
125g sugar
6 tablespoons golden syrup
250g porridge oats
A tube of Smarties

Pre-heat the oven to 180°C. Melt the butter in a medium pan over a low heat. Add the golden syrup and sugar to the butter and heat gently. Once the sugar is dissolved and the butter is melted, remove the pan from the heat and stir in the porridge oats and Smarties.

Put the flapjack mixture into a baking tin and squash down. Bake in the oven for 20 minutes, then leave to cool and cut into squares. Easy!

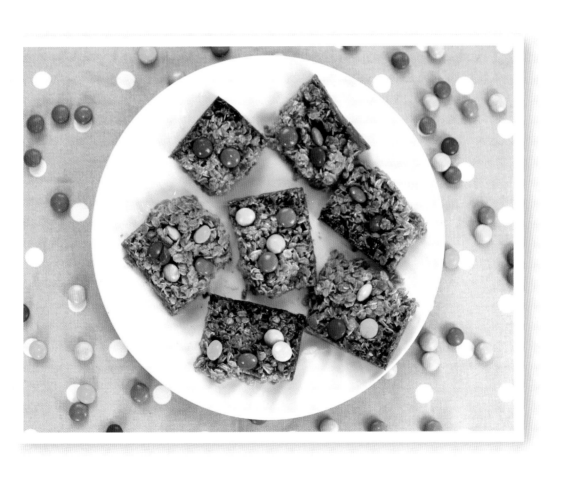

COLOURFUL DETOX JUICES

Juicing has taken over the health food world in the last couple of years and I'm always reading about the benefits of juicing. You do need a juicer to make these at home, but once you've invested in one they last for ages and they aren't too expensive. When I'm buying kitchen gadgets I don't tend to go for the most expensive option and it never seems to matter! With juicing I don't give myself loads of rules when it comes to making quantities. I just like to throw bits into the juicer and add coconut water, until I have a whole glass of juice. These are my favourite flavour combinations and I've named them after some of my best-loved Disney characters.

SIMBA

Apple, watermelon, strawberries and coconut water

This is the perfect beginner juice. If you're new to juicing, fruit-based juices are great to start off with because they are so sweet and yummy. Watermelon contains loads of Vitamin C and a nutrient called lycopene, which is important for heart and bone health, while coconut water is super-hydrating.

PETER PAN

Pineapple, spinach, cucumber, kale and coconut water

This is packed full of goodness: spinach is an excellent source of iron and many vitamins including Vitamins K, A, C and folic acid; kale is packed with antioxidants and calcium; and pineapple contains bags of fibre, thiamin and B vitamins. This juice tastes very green and when I first tried it I thought it was a bit gross, but I've grown to like it because it is so refreshing.

MALEFICENT

Beetroot, carrot, orange, ginger and strawberries

This one is the most beautiful colour and even just looking at it makes me happy! Beetroot and ginger are health food heroes – beetroot contains loads of iron, vitamins and minerals, and ginger has loads of healing properties.

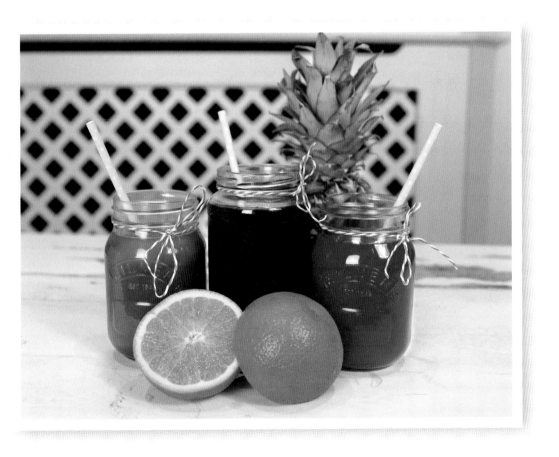

MY TOP 10
TIPS FOR SUCCESSFUL BAKING

1 | **HAVE A CLEAN KITCHEN**
Always start with a clean kitchen. You don't want to be falling over last night's dinner plates and the day's breakfast mess. I make enough mess as it is when I'm baking and I always find I need so much equipment that I need all the surfaces to be clear when I start.

2 | **GET OUT ALL OF YOUR EQUIPMENT FIRST**
Think about everything you could need before you start and get it out of the cupboards and drawers first. I always freak out halfway through my bake because I can't find the whisk!

3 | **WEIGH ALL YOUR INGREDIENTS CAREFULLY**
This is an easy thing to get right so don't just chuck everything in without measuring and weighing carefully because it can change the consistency and flavour of your bake. Follow the order of your recipe to ensure you don't miss an important ingredient out. You can also tick off ingredients as you add them if you think it will help you.

4 | **BE INSPIRED**
Whether it's watching the *Great British Bake-Off*, watching baking tutorials on YouTube, looking at recipes in your favourite cookbooks or reading posts from fab food bloggers, feel inspired by other people's recipes and try to

re-create them. I've always loved Mary Berry and look through her recipe books if I am looking for ideas. When I met her at the BAFTAs it was one of the best moments ever!

4 | DON'T RUSH IT

I like baking to be fun, relaxing and therapeutic so I never try to bake something complicated without giving myself enough time. Allow more time than you think you need because if you're in a big rush, your bake will probably end up being a bit disappointing.

5 | HAVE A COOL APRON

I love my Emma Bridgewater apron with hearts all over it. Just putting it on gets me in the mood for baking.

6 | ALWAYS LEAVE YOUR CAKE TO COOL BEFORE ICING IT

I always used to get my cake out of the oven and feel so excited about how it looked that I would ice it immediately. Ten minutes later all the icing would be melted and running down the sides, so make sure your cake is completely cool before you ice it.

7 | DON'T BE AFRAID TO GET CREATIVE

Always stick to measuring the main ingredients, like flour, sugar and butter carefully but after that get creative with your baking. I created my flapjack recipe when I found some Smarties in the kitchen and decided to throw them in. It's fun to mix things up and this is how you make your own signature dishes. If you make something unique, always make a note of what you have done so you can re-create it at a later date and don't just forget it immediately after eating!

9 | CREAM THE BUTTER BEFORE THE SUGAR

To get perfect light and fluffy buttercream, take the butter out of the fridge a few hours before your bake so it is soft, and always thoroughly cream the butter first before adding the sugar. If I forget to soften my butter first and then put it in the microwave, it melts around the edges and isn't the right consistency and I always find this affects how my cake tastes at the end!

10 | DON'T OPEN THE DOOR

You may be very tempted to look at your cake as it is baking, but if you open the door, the cold air will probably make your cake sink! Always pre-heat the oven; if you put your bake in before it has got to the right temperature it may affect the way it rises and, similarly, as you are putting it in, don't linger because it might let all the heat out.

NOTES

List the people you'd like to have dinner or eat cake with...

♡

MY TOP 10
PEOPLE I'D LIKE TO EAT CAKE
AND DRINK TEA WITH

1 | THE QUEEN
I'd love to ask the queen questions about what she gets up too, like what she eats for breakfast and what make-up she uses. In fact, I wish the queen daily vlogged so I could get to know her better!

2 | MARIO TESTINO
He is so creative and interesting and seems to be one of the world's friendliest people too. I love looking up interviews with him on YouTube – I think I would like him to be my new best friend. I am also really inspired by his work and really like his early photographs of Kate Moss – they are just beautiful.

3 | SHAKESPEARE
I'd really like to meet someone from this era and Shakespeare is the obvious person to choose. I studied his work at school and because my mum is an English teacher, I feel like I know most of his plays really well. I used to watch a lot of the old film adaptations while growing up.

4 | KURT COBAIN
I was in love with him as a teenager and his music was a huge part of those years. I loved the fact that he was so cool and seemed to view the world so differently to other people.

4 | AUDREY HEPBURN

As I've said before, she is my ultimate beauty icon and I think she would bring some real glamour to our cake eating.

5 | ROBIN WILLIAMS

He was so kind-hearted and hilarious and his smile just makes me want to laugh. I loved his films – some of my favourites are *Hook*, *Mrs Doubtfire* and *Aladdin*.

6 | JOSEPH GORDON-LEVITT

As well as being hot, he seems so sweet. As well as acting in loads of Hollywood films like *(500) Days of Summer*, *The Dark Knight Rises* and *Looper*, he makes YouTube videos, so we would have that in common and could natter on for hours.

8 | DRAKE

He is the coolest artist and his album, *Take Care*, is one of my favourites. Jim and I always sing along to his tracks as loudly as possible, so I'd be able to show him that I know all the lyrics to 'Headlines'!

9 | OLIVIA PALERMO

Olivia is so stylish and I would be able to spend the whole evening quizzing her about her amazing clothes.

10 | MAYA ANGELOU

I was so inspired by her work when I was younger. I read *I Know Why The Caged Bird Sings* when I was a teenager and it really affected me.

NOTES

List the recipes you want to try...

♡

NOTES

List your top ten favourite things to eat...

♡

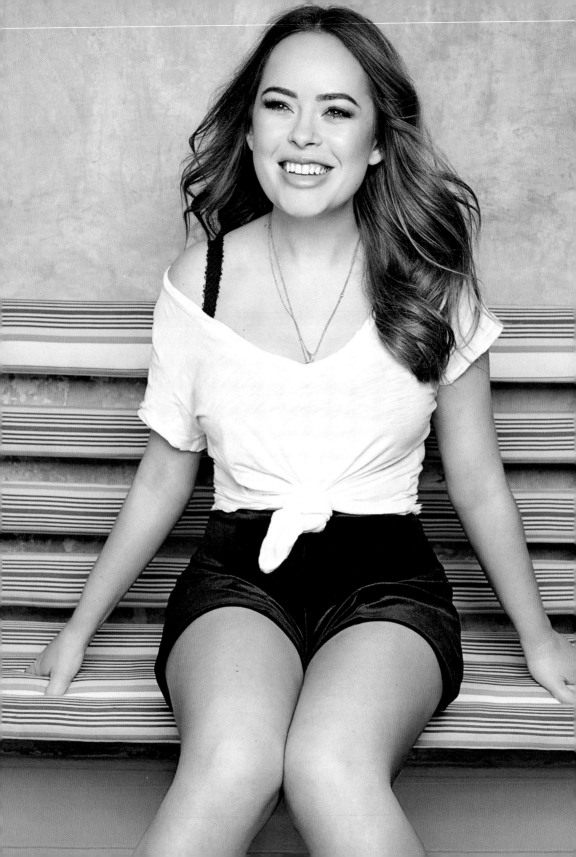

CONFIDENCE & HAPPINESS

I am so passionate that everyone should feel confident with who they are. Being confident in yourself and your abilities is one of those things that makes life better. It goes a long way, whether you're facing a difficult decision, adapting to a new situation or standing up against peer pressure, but I know it's not always that easy and it takes time.

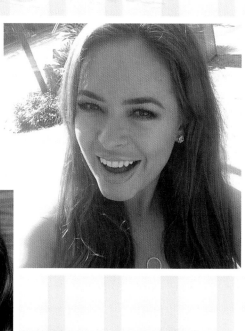

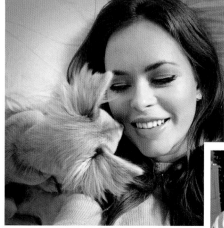

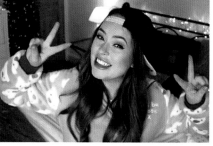

When I was younger and at high school, I found it really tough. I was so daunted by the older children and I hated it when people asked me questions or the teacher picked on me. I was really quiet and would go bright red and freeze up. Even if the rest of the class looked at me for any reason, I would feel my whole face go beetroot red from my neck upwards. It was also accompanied by this really horrible hot feeling and as soon as I knew it was happening, I just couldn't stop it. It was one of the worst things about being at school. Even in my friendship group I would hate it when all the attention was on me, like if someone told a story about me or I was put on the spot about something. It wasn't until I was about seventeen that I got over feeling like that. I think confidence can come and go depending on the situation you're in. You might be really outgoing when you're with your family and best friends but very shy at school like I was and I now realise that is completely normal.

As well as feeling confident, it is so important to feel good about your body and the way you look. As a teenager, I wanted bigger boobs like some of my friends, I hated my hair and there were some days when I hated everything about the way I looked. I also thought I was fat, which seems ridiculous looking back because I was never anything outside of completely normal. It was when I got into make-up for the first time when I was about fifteen that I started to feel better about the way I looked and this in turn made me feel more confident and happier. It meant I could experiment with my appearance and style myself like someone else. I remember that one day I was really

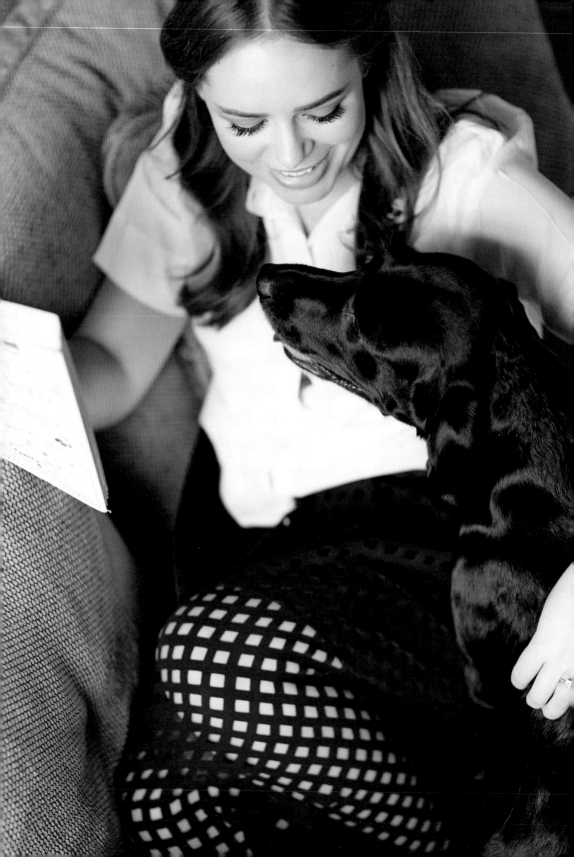

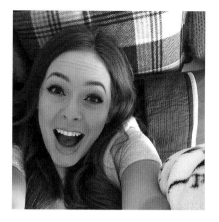

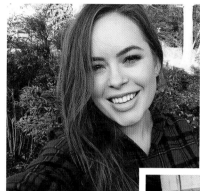

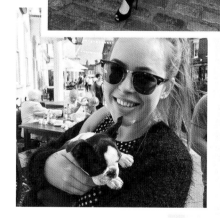

inspired by Avril Lavigne, who seemed so confident and fierce. I applied loads of black eye make-up and wore black cords, a black top and sweatbands and it made me feel really powerful and kick-ass. By doing my make-up and styling my hair in a different way, I felt so much better. I think everyone can get inspiration from someone who is confident and form an image of the person they want to be, and this really helps.

Everyone is different and confidence grows with age. Enjoy your body, your looks and your shape but remember that it's normal to feel bad sometimes, so if you don't feel great, don't give yourself a hard time. There was a time when I hated not wearing make-up and now I vlog completely barefaced, without a scrap of make-up, in front of thousands of people. Just know you are worthy and deserve to feel great.

MY TOP 10
WAYS TO FEEL MORE CONFIDENT

1 | **WALK THE WALK**
Behave as if you were someone with loads of confidence by standing tall, carrying your head high and dressing well. By doing this, you will send the signal to both yourself and others that you are capable of doing anything you set your mind to.

2 | **TALK TO FAMILY AND FRIENDS**
If you're feeling down about yourself, get your family and friends to tell you all the things they love about you. If you are worried about something specific and it is getting you down, talking to a good friend can help simplify things and put them into perspective.

3 | **FIND YOUR FASHION INSPIRATION**
Whether it's a friend, someone you go to school or work with, or a celebrity, styling yourself on a more confident person, will make you feel more optimistic. I used to always admire girls in the years above me at school and study their every move!

4 | **FACE YOUR FEARS**
By trying new things that you would normally avoid, you are stepping out of your comfort zone and making a fresh start. The rush from making these changes will boost your self-esteem. I remember being really worried about travelling to London on my own and thought I would get

lost but when I finally did it, not only did I survive
(of course!), but I also felt brilliant afterwards.

5 | **TAKE COMPLIMENTS**
Don't brush off compliments but learn to accept them.
By doing this you will help to counterbalance negative
thought patterns and build confidence.

6 | **DON'T COMPARE YOURSELF TO OTHERS**
Remember you are unique and your talents and
successes are entirely your own. It might seem like other
people have wonderful lives but we never truly know
what journey other people are on and everyone develops
at different times. One of the sayings I like is, 'Don't
overestimate everyone else and underestimate yourself.'

7 | **DON'T ALWAYS SEEK APPROVAL**
Not everyone is going to think you're great all the
time so try not to worry what other people think. The
only approval you really need is from inside yourself.

8 | **EAT, EXERCISE, PAMPER**
A good way to start feeling more confident about
who you are and what you can do is looking after yourself
physically – by eating well and exercising. Also treat
yourself to a well-deserved pamper session at least once
a week and do whatever makes you feel good, be it having
a long bubble bath, putting on a face mask or painting
your toenails.

9 | REDEFINE FAILURE

Don't ponder over your mistakes or areas in your life when you haven't achieved what you wanted to. Look at every experience as a learning one and you can't go wrong. A good example of this is if you don't get a job you want – use the interview as a learning experience, ask for feedback and move on. You never know what's around the corner!

10 | CELEBRATE YOUR ACHIEVEMENTS

Reward yourself for the things you do well. Everyone has accomplished something in their lives, no matter whether it's something huge or something tiny. Confidence will come naturally if you recognise and enjoy your successes.

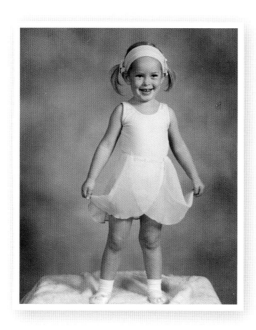

NOTES

List the things you aspire to be fearless at...

♡

MY TOP 10
THINGS THAT MAKE ME HAPPY

1 | BAKING
As you know, baking makes me feel really calm, relaxed and happy.

2 | LUSH BUBBLE BATHS
I love baths and would have one every day if I could. Some of my favourite bath products come from Lush, because they smell delicious. I enjoy the whole experience of choosing what bubbles I'm going to have, lighting candles and placing them all around the edge of the bath and just lying back with a book feeling completely chilled.

3 | PLAYING THE PIANO
I played piano up until grade six but I eventually gave up. Basically I lost interest because I was too busy being a teenager. This is one of my biggest regrets but, recently, Jim and I bought a piano for our flat and I have started playing again. If I'm learning something really difficult, I can completely lose myself in it for an hour or two.

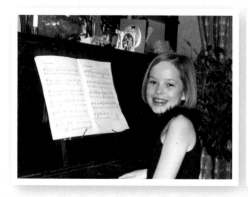

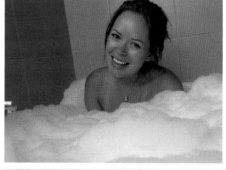

4 | THE SEA

There is something so calming and tranquil about the sea. Just sitting and watching the waves crash against the shore can be so hypnotic and relaxing.

5 | BLUE SKIES AND SUNNY DAYS

Nothing beats the feeling of being outside if the sun is shining and the skies are blue. Even if it's freezing, I will wrap up warm and it always lifts my mood. Sometimes I feel anxious when it's cloudy, but once someone told me to imagine that clear, blue sky is just above the clouds, to visualise you are on a plane and break through the clouds and picture the beautiful blue sky above it. Now if it is grey outside, I like to imagine it is a crystal-clear day.

6 | REALLY COSY PJS

I have lots and lots of pyjamas, all of which are very cosy with cute prints on them. One of my most recent buys was an incredible fluffy white dressing gown with bear ears from Topshop. It is so soft and has made me very happy.

7 | SINGING ALONG

Whether it's to Disney or Beyoncé, singing along to my favourite tracks is a guaranteed way of making me feel cheerful.

8 | FIREWORKS

I think everything about Guy Fawkes night is magical. I love being wrapped up warm with a sparkler in my hand and watching the sky in anticipation as the pretty fireworks illuminate the sky.

9 | HAVING A CUP OF TEA AND WATCHING *THE VAMPIRE DIARIES*

If I have time, I like to take an hour's break in the day ` to have a cup of tea in one of my favourite mugs and watch *The Vampire Diaries* on Netflix. It's one of my guilty pleasures. I often do it in between filming and editing and when I come back to work, I feel relaxed and content.

10 | CHARBONNEL ET WALKER CHOCOLATES

There is something really special about a beautiful box of chocolates and I love the packaging of Charbonnel et Walker goodies. I always keep the boxes for their sentimental value.

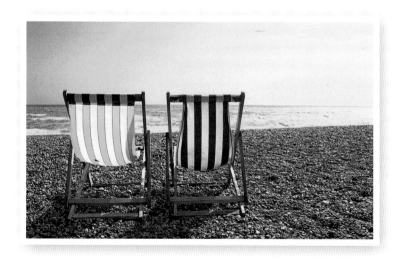

NOTES

List the things that make you happy...

- -

- -

- -

- -

- -

- -

- -

- -

- -

- -

- -

- -

- -

- -

- -

- -

♡

ANXIETY AND STRESS

Since I was a teenager I have suffered from anxiety and panic attacks. Some people say to me, 'How can you have anxiety when you have such a great life and go to premieres and stuff like that?' But for me, doing these kind of things doesn't change the fact that I might have days where I feel really stressed and overwhelmed. Many people suffer from anxiety and different mental health conditions on loads of different levels and it is a huge topic, but some of my viewers have said that knowing I have suffered with anxiety has helped them. If you are one of these people, I hope that by talking about it and telling you how I stay positive and knowing that you're not alone, comforts you in some way.

Everyone suffers from some level of anxiety and worries over things like school exams or problems at work because it's a normal emotional state, but once the difficult situation is over, they feel calmer. Some people have an abnormal amount of anxiety and feel fearful when there's nothing to be anxious about and this is when it becomes a problem and can affect their everyday lives. Panic can sometimes be like a bit of a vicious cycle because the fear of your life spinning out of control often leads to you feeling even more anxious.

According to research, it is said that one in four people will suffer from some form of mental health problem within their lives, and a large percentage of these problems will be related to anxiety or depression. So even if someone seems perfectly happy on the outside, you

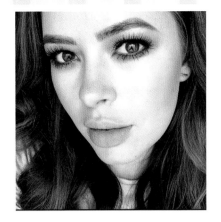

never know what's going on inside their head. Each person's struggle is totally unique to them. For example, although my friend Zoe and I can relate to each other a lot as she also experiences anxiety, the things that make us panic are totally different. I've never liked talking about it but I've actually found it easier to open up and speak about my experiences with anxiety as I've become older because I have realised that so many people suffer with it in some shape or form. A handful of people I work with do, and even members of my family and good friends have struggled with it on occasion. I think it's important to talk, yet not focus on the bad times, and to look forward to how you can make things better.

For me I find my anxiety easiest to describe as feeling unsettled and a horrible feeling of dread. Sometimes the unsettled feeling can lead to a panic attack, caused by a sudden rush of adrenaline and an uncontrollable level of anxiety; my heart starts hammering and I feel sick and faint. This is a side of me that is very different to the one that most people see in my videos, when I am very happy and smiley. Of course I'm not really anxious all the time. On the whole I am a really positive, bubbly, happy person, but I have my ups and downs just like everyone else and my downs are usually related to the fact that I sometimes struggle with anxiety. The scariest part for me was when I was younger, as I didn't speak to anyone about it properly and I felt totally isolated and thought I was going crazy. It totally ruined my self-esteem. When I was about fourteen

I couldn't sleep or eat properly for months. My parents tried to help and a therapist came to the house but I wasn't ready to speak about it. I was so confused and thought I was crazy, so I just blocked her out. I remember coming down from upstairs in my house where I had been having a bath and I sat on the sofa and didn't listen to a word she said. Since then I have learned more about myself and how to manage my anxiety. I have come to accept that when I feel anxious, sometimes it lasts for days and sometimes for weeks. Most of the time I feel so great and happy that when it happens it knocks me sideways, but it comes and goes and I've learned to deal with it better.

Talking to a therapist I was recommended to see has been life-changing for me. It had got to a point where I felt trapped in most situations and it was making my everyday life very difficult because I was making decisions based on my anxiety. Not only has she helped me to work on my fears and worries but she's also made me become aware and mindful of the influence that my day-to-day thoughts have on my life and has taught me lots of different coping mechanisms; she's also taught me to work with my thoughts rather than resist them. We have done some hypnosis, which is a pleasant state of deep relaxation and enhanced awareness.

Just a few months after I started working with her, I started feeling much better. She also says things to me like, 'Be kinder to yourself, it starts with you.' The change in me didn't happen overnight. When I first started seeing my therapist it took me three months to feel better and get on top of my feelings. She has helped me see that I need balance in my life. When I am crazily busy and I don't sleep enough or give myself time for just me, I am more prone to feeling anxious. There was a time when I had something on every hour of every day, but I don't pack my diary so full any more. I know many people work long hours but my work also keeps going, so I always try to give myself a quiet day once a week where I can work on my blog or catch up on personal stuff.

However, too much time off and nothing to do can also make me feel anxious. My life has been very hectic for a few years but when I left school and was working part time, sometimes I felt a bit directionless and would feel anxious. I think everyone should apply this idea about balance to their lives; keep busy, have fun, work hard and go out as much as you like but don't overdo it. If you're between jobs or have a long period of time with nothing planned, make a plan to make the most of your time. I like to treat myself like one of those characters from The Sims, where players must fulfil their need to sleep, eat, acquire knowledge and so on, just like real human beings, and you can tell because they have these bars that show the different areas in their lives. There was one time when my sister and I were playing and we left our characters to go off and have dinner or something. When we came back, they were going mental and crying because their bars were low. Now I like to think of myself and other people like that and I think that being happy is all about balance. I like to keep the levels in different areas of my life well balanced, and as well as making sure I eat well and sleep enough, I spend time with my family and friends and keep stimulated intellectually.

Another thing I find helps me when I'm feeling anxious is being distracted and having something else to focus on. Recently Jim and I were in a taxi and I started to feel bad, so we made up this whole story, using loads of different characters from various ages throughout history – it was a bit bonkers but it stopped me from thinking too much about how I was feeling and my anxiety really subsided.

Sometimes I struggle to sleep at night because I have so many thoughts whizzing around my head, but I've learned ways of making myself relax. For a start I make sure I switch off all my electronic devices, like my phone and my laptop, and take them out of the room because the light affects the body's natural rhythms by releasing a hormone called cortisol, which makes us feel more awake. This hormone is also released in response to stress. I make sure I start to wind down at least an hour before bedtime and I tidy and potter around my bedroom, turn on my fairy lights, spray some This Works Deep Sleep Pillow spray onto my pillow and relax with a book. I find that reading really helps to focus my mind and switch off other worries and that after reading for a while, my eyelids will feel tired and heavy.

Now, I feel like I can handle so many situations I wouldn't have been able to manage a couple of years ago. I'm also feeling anxious a lot less, which is so great. I have seen therapists on and off since I was about thirteen, but had never stuck with one before; I would just do the odd session and expect it to work first time. All I can say is that if you suffer from anxiety try to stick with working on it. I am so, so happy that I did and I wish you the best of luck. Obviously my therapist has helped me massively, so if you are struggling with anxiety please tell someone, whether it's a doctor, friend or parent, and make sure you find someone who can really help you, even if that means trying a couple of different therapists – just please don't feel alone.

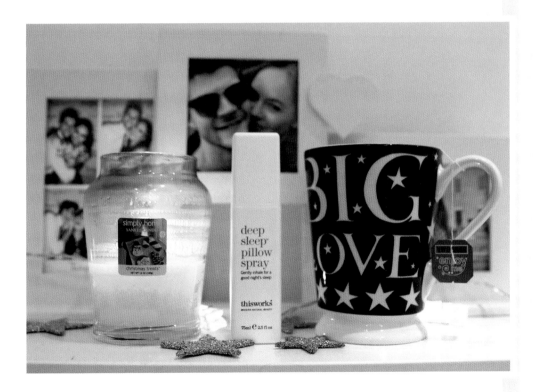

MY TOP 10
WAYS OF DEALING WITH ANXIETY AND STRESS

1 | USE CALMING TECHNIQUES

I use a calming technique my therapist taught me called 'The five Stages Of The Sea'. You can do it anywhere, even on the bus. Close your eyes and imagine a really stormy, wild sea at night, with thunder and lightning in the sky. Unsurprisingly, this image is really easy to conjure up when you're feeling really stressed. Then imagine the sea and sky starting to calm down, and at each stage, imagine it calming down more and more, until it's dawn the next day and the sea is still, the sky is clear and bright and the only noise you hear is a seagull passing by. I always find that by this time, I feel much more calm and centred. This is just one example of lots of different techniques that you can use.

2 | FIND SOMETHING THAT IS A COMFORT TO YOU

Personally, I sometimes get anxious when I am travelling, so I like to take something which connects me to home. When I went away recently, I packed one of my favourite mugs and my Disney blanket and it really made a difference having those things with me.

3 | ASK YOURSELF 'WHAT IF?'

When I'm stressed and feeling anxious, I ask myself 'What if?' about whatever I'm worrying about. I then think of the worst possible outcome, which is never normally all that bad, and if I'm still anxious I continue to ask myself the same question until it feels better in my head.

4 | YOGA

Yoga is brilliant for making sure you take long, deep breaths and focus on the present moment. By observing your breath, it can make such a difference to how you feel. I think sometimes it is easy to not stop and actually focus on breathing properly. Yoga is great for practising slowly taking breaths in through your nose and out through your mouth.

5 | REMEMBER THAT IT WILL PASS

I think this is one of the most important things that I learned, that how I'm feeling will pass. I remind myself that when I'm feeling bad, it will pass because nobody has ever been stuck in the exact same emotional state for ever. No matter how anxious I'm feeling, I know I won't feel the same in a few hours, or the next day.

6 | DO SIMPLE THINGS

I do simple things like relax in a warm bubble bath and read a book. Never underestimate how valuable time on your own, caring for yourself, can be.

7 | LISTEN TO MUSIC

Music can lift your mood and help you to think positively. The music you listen to doesn't necessarily have to be about how great life is, just songs you enjoy. At the moment when I'm feeling stressed, I like to listen to Ed Sheeran.

8 | MEDITATE

I use www.calm.com where you can do guided meditations for two, five, ten, fifteen or twenty minutes. Even if I just meditate for two minutes, I find this really helps to put things in perspective.

9 | USE POSITIVE AFFIRMATIONS

I use positive affirmations and quotes to help me feel stronger and remind me to think positively. I have lots written down, some I've found in books and online and some I've made up (a little tip is to only make up your positive affirmations when you are in a positive mind-set; don't try and do it when you're already feeling anxious or down as you'll find it much harder). It's incredible how much of a difference a few words can make if you really listen to them. Here are two things I say to myself a lot: 'Be bright. Be happy. Be you' and 'You're stronger than you think'.

10 | TRY AND STAY IN THE MOMENT

Don't fret too much about things that are happening in the future. Take each day as it comes and try to focus on this moment in time.

NOTES

*List the things to make yourself feel better
when you're feeling down...*

♡

MY FAVOURITE INSPIRATIONAL QUOTES

'You have to be odd to be number one.'

'Don't be afraid to be different.'

'The greatest act of courage is to be and own all that you are. Without apology. Without excuses and without any masks to cover the truth of who you really are.'

'You're stronger than you think.'

'Success is liking yourself, liking what you do and liking how you do it.'

'If you're always trying to be normal, you'll never know how amazing you can be.'

'Life is better when you're laughing.'

'Today I choose happiness.'

'Be a warrior not a worrier.'

'Dream BIG.'

'Don't fill your head with worries –
there won't be room for anything else!'

'Don't worry about things that haven't
happened yet.'

'Wake up and live.'

'One small positive thought in the morning
can change your whole day.'

'Every day is an adventure.'

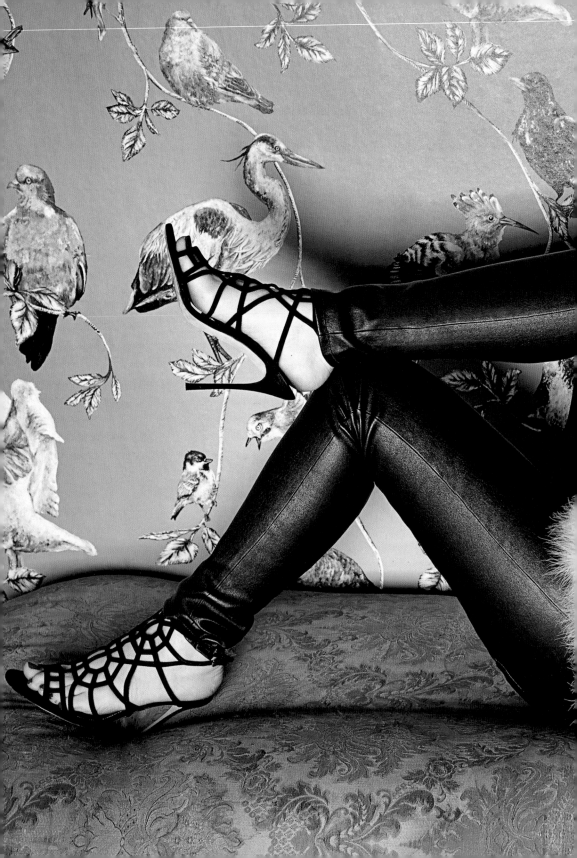

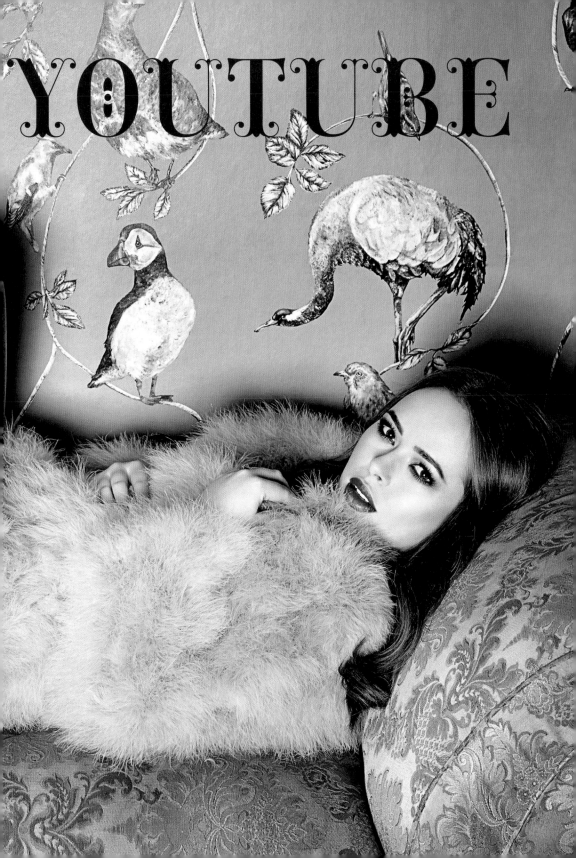

From when I was quite young, computers have been part of
my life. I always had a desktop PC in my room at home and
I used computers for school and for writing my homework.
Outside of schoolwork, other than MSN Messenger, which
I used to chat to all my friends after school, I used to look
at celebrity style on magazine sites and check out MySpace
too. When I was about twelve or thirteen, I was obsessed
with Sienna Miller and I always used to tear pictures out of
magazines of her walking her dog and wearing cool cowboy
boots and boho dresses. Before I started uploading videos to
YouTube, I never looked at YouTube or other people's blogs.

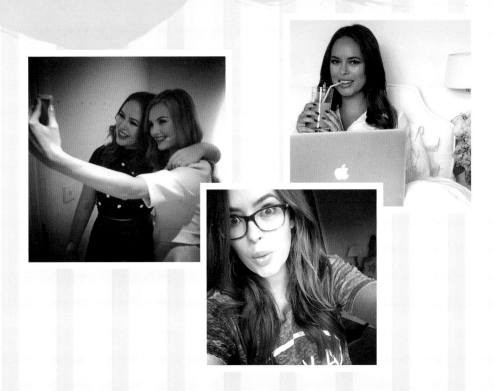

When I started posting my videos to YouTube, it was just a creative outlet for me and it was almost by accident that they became really successful. I started by doing make-up tutorials and used it as a creative outlet; I had no idea it could be a career or a business. My first video was a make-up tutorial recreating the look of Serena van der Woodsen from *Gossip Girl*, who was played by Blake Lively. When I started uploading videos, they were almost always tutorials inspired by the looks of younger celebrities, such as Hilary Duff and Emma Watson. I usually looked for inspiration from TV shows I was watching back then, like *Gossip Girl* or *The X Factor*, or the style of pop stars in music videos.

When I look back, I think I appear so shy and awkward. The one thing I have always loved from the start was the interaction with the viewers and I have always been fascinated by what people say about my videos. Back then, the quality was really poor and I used Jim's MacBook for a year before I bought my own. When I got back from travelling and started doing my tutorials in HD, it was really fun because I could actually see what I was doing!

A turning point for me came when I realised I needed to put more personality into my videos. On our return from mine and Jim's travels, I wanted to do more make-up tutorials, but think I had a newfound confidence and was more chatty and personable. Viewers started commenting on how they liked to see my personality and the way I chatted more about general stuff, like my day or sharing anecdotes. I had grown quite a big audience by this point and I think they felt like they were really getting to know me, almost like you get to know a friend. Sometimes I would get stopped in the street; in fact the first time I ever got stopped on the street was when we were travelling in Sydney. I was walking down George Street and I heard someone shout my name. I was so confused because I knew that none of my friends were out there but it turned out that it was one of my Australian viewers. She looked quite embarrassed and like she hadn't meant to shout at me, and it felt crazy to know that someone on the other side of the world had been watching my tutorials.

With the comments from my viewers saying they wanted to get to know more about other parts of my life, not just the make-up, I sometimes did the odd video where I started rambling on about different stuff and goofing around doing daily vlogs. Videos are different from vlogs because in traditional videos, the camera is fixed and you sit or stand in front of it, whereas with vlogs I took the camera out with me and took loads of footage of where I was going, what I was doing, and talked about whatever was going on that day. They are very personality driven but fun and easy to make and I found that I didn't need to be doing anything particularly special to engage with my viewers. It was almost like having a friendly chat with one of my friends about what I was going to make for lunch. The vlogs were really popular and made my number of subscribers shoot up. I love vlogging because it makes me feel like I am sharing my everyday life.

For someone who wants to start vlogging or uploading videos to YouTube, I think the real key is to do something you are interested in. So for me, I was passionate about beauty and decided to start with that. I think it's so

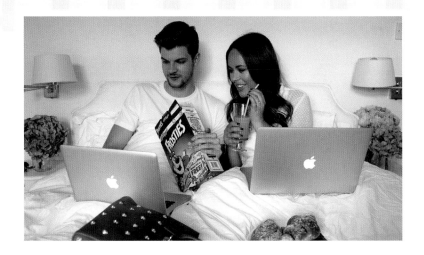

important to put your whole personality into videos. When I first started I used to say in a serious voice, 'You need to put contour here and blush here', and I never put my true self into the videos because I still felt quite shy. I have learned that this is one of the most important things to do because your personality is what people come back for. Let it shine through! I don't think it matters at all if there are other vloggers doing the same thing or covering the same topics because everyone is unique.

Many of my YouTube friends like Zoe, Louise and Ruth cover beauty and fashion like me, but I think of their videos as completely different. There is room for everyone! For me, it reminds me of when you are young and like looking at the older girl at school to see how she does her hair or picks her clothes out. I always watch the channels of people I am interested in and inspired by.

When I first started, I only had my laptop and I did everything on there, so you don't need to buy expensive equipment or products to start vlogging. Also, you don't need to do anything special. Some of the best videos are of someone making their tea and breakfast in the morning. I think it's important to not think too hard about it because if you do that you start to censor yourself too much.

At the beginning, I just saw YouTube as a little, fun project. I think if you are starting out, then don't become too obsessed with worrying about how many people are watching because if people like you, your viewer base will naturally follow.

Social media is really important when you're posting videos and I can't express how important it is to share your videos through platforms like Twitter and Facebook. It's also important to upload content that you think other people will want to share, because you need other people to share it too in order for your brand to grow. I started my YouTube channel first, and then I put up my blog because I thought it looked fun and would be a good chance for me to post some of my pictures. Around the same time, I started on Facebook and Twitter and then set up my Instagram account later. I like to keep some of my content exclusive to one platform to keep it interesting and so that people have a reason to visit each one.

I love the fact that my videos appeal to people in different countries, all over the world. Some of my strongest fan bases are in America, Canada, Germany, Ireland, Sweden, Netherlands, France and New Zealand, and one of my favourite things is going to meet-and-greets in different countries. Also, even if I'm awake in the middle of the night, there will be someone in a different time zone to talk to. I love being part of such an amazing online community.

Here are my top tips for making videos and putting them online:

DO

★ Be yourself: people watch other people online mainly because they like their personalities and want to know more about them. Even if, like me, you start off with beauty tutorials, offer up anecdotes about your day or something that has happened or a memory, to help people get to know you. So when applying eyeliner, talk about the day you went to buy it and how you tried the new drink at Starbucks, for example.

★ Be an expert but vary your content: find your niche, your main interest – and your unique selling point! Mine is mostly beauty and fashion. I love that my fans see me as their go-to girl for tips, tricks and trends. However, at the same time, vary your content to show the different elements of your personality. I love filming my baking videos and doing 'day in the life' vlogs.

★ Listen to your audience and interact with your viewers: it's really important to listen to what your audience wants but, at the same time, don't lose your focus so that you find yourself moving away from topics you are passionate about because your viewers might be asking about something else.

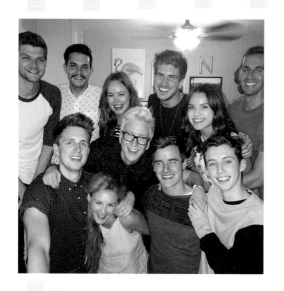

★ Keep your tweets interesting: don't make all your tweets about promoting your YouTube video or asking people to subscribe to your channel. People are interested in your opinions and love to ask questions.

★ Keep up with the latest social media trends: right now, the latest social media craze is SnapChat and to be successful online it's important to know what people are excited about and talking about. For me, another big thing at the moment is daily vlogging, where I post a video every day. It's hard work but when I did it in September 2014, over the course of the month my videos had more views than I've ever had in a single month.

★ Network with other bloggers: I think it's really nice to build relationships with other people, bloggers or Youtubers because you can share tips and experiences.

★ Be proud of your YouTube channel: never be embarrassed about any videos you have uploaded or blogs you have written. If your friends at school or work find out about it, be proud!

DON'T

★ Pay attention to negative comments: unless ninety-five per cent of your comments are asking you to do something like stop saying 'um' all the time, in which case maybe you do need to think about it, don't pay attention to horrible comments. There are always people online who aren't going to like everything about what you do.

★ Stress over statistics and views: I said it before, but try not to worry about how many people are watching your videos at the beginning; it takes a long, long time to build a solid viewer base. However, while I don't believe you should obsess over stats too much, it's a good idea to keep on top of them because this can help you stay focused and you can make adjustments based on these numbers so that your videos and blogs are the best they can be.

★ Be a copycat: by all means be inspired by other people's blogs and videos and borrow their ideas, but don't try and analyse too closely or copy what other people are doing.

★ Be afraid to hit 'publish': there have been some vlogs that I have felt nervous about uploading, like one last September where I felt really anxious, but actually it got some great responses and made me feel much better. If you're honest and open, I think the response will always be positive.

★ Feel like you have to vlog or blog every day: sometimes I am just so busy with work, which means I can't post videos or blogs as much as I would like. However, when you start out it is really important to be consistent, so whether you post a daily blog or a weekly video, try to keep it regular for a while so that your viewers know what to expect.

★ Compare yourself to others: don't compare your life with someone else's highlights. When you're looking online a lot it can feel like everyone's Instagram is amazing, but the truth is you never really know what is going on in someone else's life – people don't share the less glamorous stuff!

NOTES

List your top ten favourite websites...

- -
- -
- -
- -
- -
- -
- -
- -
- -
- -
- -
- -
- -
- -

♡

MY TOP 10
VLOGGING AND BLOGGING
TIPS FOR BEGINNERS

1 | **USE NATURAL LIGHT**
Always try to shoot your videos in natural light because that's how they will look their best, unless you have a lighting system.

2 | **HAVE A PLAN**
Although I am known for never getting to the point (!), have a plan beforehand so you know what you are going to say and do, otherwise you could end up filming a ramble that is pretty hard to follow.

3 | **MIX IT UP**
Mix up your content so you have some videos that will make people laugh and others that are more serious and informative.

4 | **TEACH YOURSELF HOW TO EDIT**
I taught myself how to edit videos on iMovie and how to take good pictures and have just got better as time's gone on. Google is your best friend!

5 | **TAKE YOUR TIME**
Don't expect your first video or blog post to be perfect. Give yourself a bit of time to improve and never rush what you are doing. Even if it means getting up an hour earlier to do some filming or writing, this is better than rushing the process.

6 | EDIT LATER

With blog posts, it is really reassuring to remember that you can edit them later. With one of my recipes for cookies, I made them at a later date and added the new pictures because the second batch looked much better!

7 | MAKE IMAGES INTERESTING

When taking photos for your blog, think of it in terms of lighting, colours and setting. If you are taking pictures of a candle for example, don't feel like you just have to have the candle in the shot but fill the background of the picture with pretty things, like fresh flowers or a stack of cute notepads, for extra interest.

8 | DON'T FOCUS ON STATS

Remember that building a viewer base takes time. It's important to be patient; so many people give up too quickly because they don't see instant results. Have fun, let your personality shine through and the viewers will follow!

9 | KEEP IT NORMAL

Don't think that you always need to have something fun to do. Walking to the shop to buy some milk can make a really fun vlog. Not everyone has exciting activities planned every day.

10 | REMEMBER THE PICTURES

If you are writing a blog, don't publish large chunks of text without breaking it up with pictures. I love photos so much – they really do speak a thousand words.

MY TOP 10
MOMENTS OF MY YOUTUBE CAREER SO FAR

I've had so many incredible experiences since starting my YouTube channel and it is so hard to pick the best ones, but here goes:

1 | MY FIRST-EVER MEET-AND-GREET

I did my first ever meet-and-greet at the Starbucks on Vigo Street in London in March 2011. I was really nervous in case no one turned up and thought I might be drinking my coffee on my own, so I made Kate come with me. It was a really last-minute thing because I was going to be in London for a fashion event and when I realised I had an hour free beforehand, I thought it would be the perfect opportunity; I just picked a venue nearby and made a video. About twenty people came along and I just loved meeting some of my viewers and getting some feedback. I have loved every meet-and-greet event since – they are always one of my big highlights.

2 | SITTING ON THE FROW AT MULBERRY

Mulberry has been a brand that I have loved for years and I have built a relationship with them. I was lucky enough to sit on the front row of the spring/summer 2014 show in September 2013 alongside Alexa Chung and Douglas Booth. The show always has a special feel about it and this one in particular because it was creative director Emma Hill's last collection for the brand.

Emma did such a fantastic job at Mulberry creating such stunning looks for six years. I wore head-to-toe Mulberry for the first time, as they dressed me for the show, which was such an amazing experience!

3 | GOING TO *THE HUNGER GAMES: CATCHING FIRE* PREMIERE

In November 2013, I was invited to attend *The Hunger Games: Catching Fire* world premiere in Leicester Square and I was thrilled to be asked. I was feeling super-glamorous that night; I was wearing a full-length dress from Coast, had my hair up in pretty braids and my friend Adam had done my make-up. As I stepped onto the red carpet with my friend Maddie, all the photographers were shouting my name. It was also crazy because there were so many of my viewers on the red carpet, which I totally wasn't expecting! I spent about an hour having my photo taken with loads of them. It was such a buzz and after watching the film, we were lucky enough to go to the after-party at the Royal Courts of Justice!

It was the coolest party and the food was amazing – banquet tables piled high with all sorts of gorgeous food like salted caramel profiteroles and old-fashioned pick'n'mix sweeties. The venue was beautiful and it really reminded me of Hogwarts. There were these incredible pink cocktails in martini glasses with popping candy around the edge. I took so many photos!

4 | YOUTUBERS TRIP TO DUBAI

In December 2013, I went to Dubai to film a look-book for a YouTube channel called Daily Mix with Zoe, Alfie, Jim, Joe, Ruth, Niomi and Marcus. I hate not working but I love a 'working holiday' and this was the perfect combination of work and play. We stayed at the Atlantis, The Palm hotel and spent a lot of time lying on sun-loungers and drinking cocktails. I had been to Dubai before and done all the touristy stuff, so while some of the others left the resort, I stayed there and hung out at the spa and on the beach.

5 | ATTENDING THE BAFTAS

Usually I wouldn't be allowed to go to the BAFTAs because I'm not an actress, obviously (although that sounds like such an awesome job!), but I have been kindly invited to go for the last couple of years by the hair brand Charles Worthington, who are official sponsors. On both occasions, it was such a special and magical evening. Last year, the part I enjoyed most was hearing the directors' speeches about their stories behind the films. After the awards there was a dinner and it felt very surreal sitting eating dinner in the same room as George Clooney, Angelina Jolie and Brad Pitt! I had some lovely people on my table from Charles Worthington, and also Sai Bennett from the ITV show *Mr Selfridge* and Samantha Barks from the musical *Les Miserables*. None of us knew one another, but we had such a fun evening together.

6 | BEING NAMED AS ONE OF *GQ*'S 100 MOST CONNECTED WOMEN

In September 2014, I was named as one of GQ magazine's Most Connected Women. I was listed under the 'Influencer' category and the list contained so many amazing women, like Stella McCartney, Anya Hindmarsh, Victoria Beckham, Jessica Ennis-Hill and Tracey Emin, to name just a few. It was such an incredible honour and I still can't quite believe it.

7 | LAUNCHING MY TANYA BURR COSMETICS RANGE

As well as my nail polishes and lip glosses, which launched in January 2014, more recently I launched a range of false eyelashes. The party was held last October at the Sanderson Hotel again and it was brilliant. All my favourite people were there and it was packed out with press and guests. I spent half the night in the photo booth with all my friends and family pulling ridiculous faces and my dad even had some of my individual lashes applied to show his support! All my family and Jim had written me really cute cards saying well done, including one from Oscar where he had drawn some cartoon eyelashes on.

8 | AMITY FEST

In October 2014, we went on the Amity Fest tour. We do so many events but they are never exactly how we want them because we're not in control, so we decided to set up our own tour, called Amity Fest. Jim and I, Zoe, Alfie, Niomi, Marcus, Louise and Caspar all participated and we performed at venues in Brighton, Liverpool and

Birmingham. Sadly Joe was ill for the first two nights so we took a cardboard cut-out of him on stage with us, but halfway through the Brighton show he came on stage and kicked it down – I was so shocked to see him! It was completely sold out and the atmosphere was electric every night. We also did some meet-and-greets before each show and normally they feel so rushed, so it was really good to meet our viewers in such a relaxed environment.

9 | BEING AN AMBASSADOR FOR CHILDREN IN NEED

In October 2014, I was honoured to take part in the BearFaced campaign to raise funds and awareness for BBC's Children In Need, alongside other names including Michelle Keegan, Sophie Ellis-Bextor, Olivia Coleman and Rochelle Humes. The campaign was shot by one of my favourite photographers of all time, Rankin, who was so charming. I didn't have a scrap of make-up on but I had my hair done, which made me feel slightly more glamorous. When he took the photos, Rankin had a massive team of people holding lights around him and the results were incredible. I had loads of lovely tweets and texts when the photos were released. It felt brilliant to be involved in such a great campaign for such a fantastic cause.

10 | THIS BOOK

I've always had my nose in a book since a really young age and they are such an important part of my life, so I am incredibly excited to be writing my own. I couldn't be more excited!

NOTES

List your proudest moments...

♡

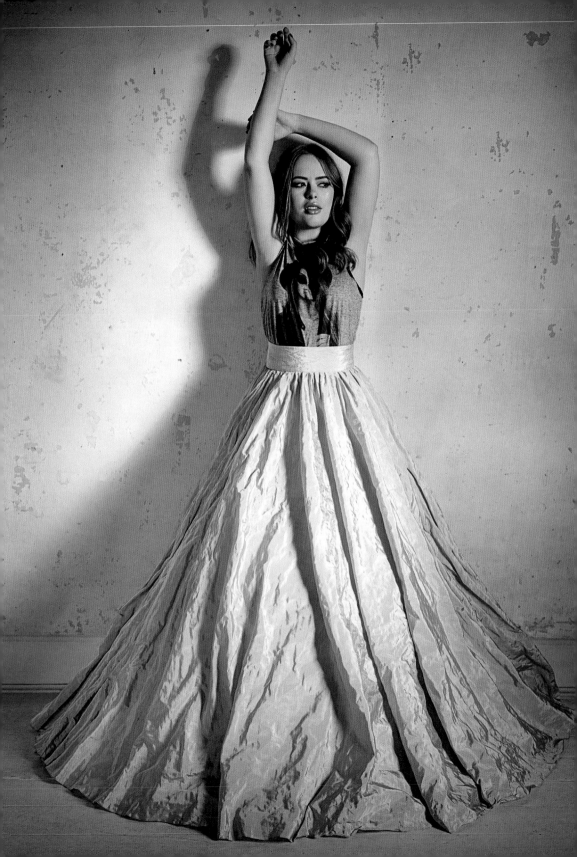

LOOKING FORWARDS

I love thinking about the future and what it might hold and writing lists about the things I want to do and achieve. At the moment, work is my number one priority and I have a real passion for what I do. As well as making videos and writing my blog, I enjoy working with some brilliant brands, being involved with some seriously cool projects and continuing to expand my Tanya Burr Cosmetics line. I have no idea what will be coming next, but I love the idea of doing a brow product or a fragrance. I have a few fragrances that I have always worn, but the one I would label as my signature scent is Chanel Chance Eau Fresh. It's a really fresh, light scent and it lasts on my skin for a long time. It would be incredible to create a scent and learn about the process of matching different scent notes together. I am also the biggest fan of scented candles and always have them burning at home, so in the future at some point I would love to design a line of candles. Some of my favourites come from Jo Malone and Diptyque.

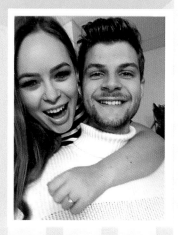

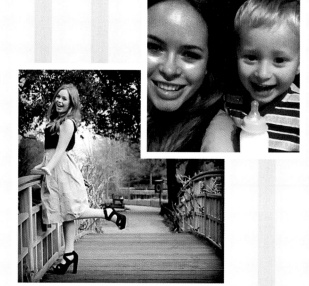

It felt like a real honour to be asked to be involved in the recent project with Children In Need and I'd love to do more for charity. I feel really privileged to be able to help and feel passionately about being able to make a difference through my influence on social media.

Life for Jim and I seems to be a crazy whirlwind of work and travel at the moment. We are so lucky that some of our work overlaps and we get to be together on some shoots, meet-and-greets or projects that we are working on. I love having him by my side, but it's also amazing that we have our own independent businesses too and can go a week without seeing each other, then have loads to talk about.

The wedding is later this year, so by the time you are reading this I hope to have more planned and looking beyond that, I'd love to have a family at some point. In my head I hope to work hard for the next five years and then have children when I am about thirty. Children might come before then, but that's my plan so far! I think I'll always want to have a career and continue working but, like my mum, I'd like to spend as much time as possible with my children. Jim and I have always said that we'd like to have children; I'd love to have a boy and a girl. I've loved watching my sister's son Isaac grow up and Sam and Nic's children, Lily, Ollie, Harry and Edie. When I met Jim, Oscar was five and just out of that baby phase and Sam's daughter Lily was one. Since then, there have always been new little people to cuddle and play with. Maybe by the time they are all grown up, it will be mine and Jim's turn!

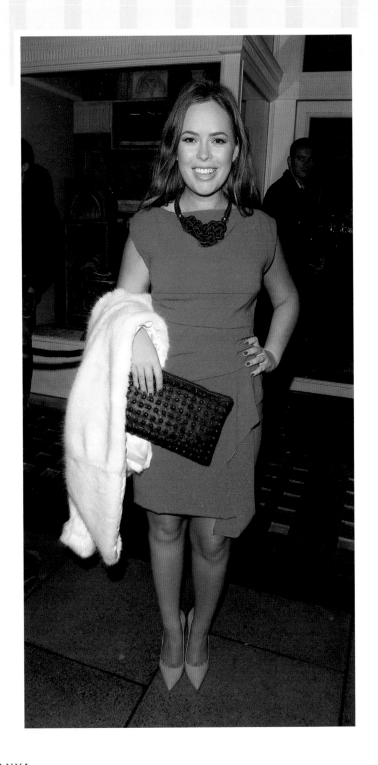

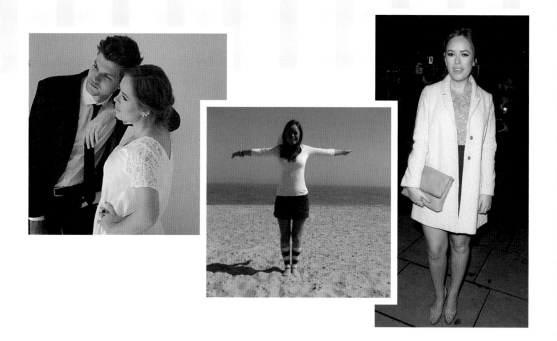

When it comes to giving career advice, I always say to do what you love. In that way hopefully you'll find something that truly reflects you, your creativity and what matters to you in life. I consider myself very lucky to have found a job that I love but for many people it takes a long time to find their niche. If you're unsure about what path to take, think about what you are good at, what you enjoy, jobs that relate to your hobbies or the things that excite you most in life. If you are stuck on the things you are good at, ask your closest friends and family or a teacher or mentor, what they think you excel at. If you try something and it doesn't work out, it doesn't matter; simply move on. Get everything you can from a job – even when I worked at Starbucks, I tried to get as much as I could from it, like learning how to work around other people, dealing with stressful situations and with the public. There is something to be learned from every job. If you follow your heart and think creatively, you will succeed!

MY TOP 10
WAYS TO GET WHAT
YOU WANT IN LIFE

1 | DREAM BIG

Allow yourself to dream big and imagine and fantasise about all your career goals and the kind of life you would like to live. Imagine you have no limitations on what you can be, have or do in life and create a vision for your long-term future. Once you have a clear vision of the life you want to achieve, then it becomes easier to take steps towards it. Jim really struggles with this idea because he is such a realist, so I always write him little notes saying things like, 'Dream Big!'

2 | BRAINSTORM

If you are unhappy with something in your life but you can't quite put your finger on why, sit down with a friend and talk to them about it. As you chat, write a list of areas in your life that you don't feel totally satisfied with and ways you might be able to improve it. Issues like not being happy at work or with your housemates might arise, or it might be something as simple as not wanting to watch so much television. By writing it down, it will then become much clearer in your mind.

3 | FOCUS ONE HUNDRED PER CENT ON YOUR GOAL

Whether your goal is health, relationship or career-related or just about simple self-fulfilment, once you have decided to do it, be committed – write it down and put it somewhere where you will see it a lot, like on your bedroom wall. Tell your friends and family what you are doing because they can offer support and encouragement and you are less likely to quit.

4 | ONLY TRY TO ACHIEVE ONE GOAL AT A TIME

If you start with a whole load of goals, you are unlikely to maintain focus and energy and manage to do all of them, so do one thing at a time. Also, if your goal is a big one, start out with a series of smaller goals. For example, if you need to get out of bed two hours earlier every day, start by setting your alarm ten minutes earlier and then twenty minutes earlier, until you reach your goal time. If you want to cut sugar out of your diet, start gradually, so if you normally have two chocolate bars a day, cut down to one, then one every other day, then one every three days and so on.

5 | BELIEVE IN YOURSELF

Everyone has the ability to believe in themselves and achieve incredible things in life. Believing in yourself is key to almost everything you might start, so if you want to start a business, not only do you need to feel passionately about what you do, you also need to believe in the fact it can work. If I want something, I like to close my eyes and imagine it happening and I find this really helps.

6 | BE PREPARED TO WORK HARD

Always be prepared to work hard and put negative thoughts out of your mind. Making changes or achieving something you may have dreamed about for a while might not be easy, but if you work hard, you can get there.

7 | DON'T BE DISCOURAGED BY SETBACKS

Everyone faces setbacks from time to time and you might be tempted to give up and ignore all the hard work you have put in to something, but remember the saying, 'One step forwards, two steps back'. Keep moving forwards.

8 | TAKE ADVANTAGE OF OPPORTUNITIES

If you're waiting for things to be perfect in your life, you might be waiting a long time – after all, nobody has the perfect life! Take advantage of every opportunity that is thrown your way and embrace it. Say yes to invitations and be prepared to take risks.

9 | BE PASSIONATE ABOUT YOUR GOAL

Look at your reasons for wanting to achieve something. You have to be passionate about it. Whatever it is, you've got to make sure you really, really want it, otherwise you might not manage it. For example, if you are being pushed down a certain career path by your parents, this might not make you very happy if you don't love the subject.

10 | ALWAYS PLAN

I write lists for everything. Every once in a while I do a career plan, so I can work out what I see happening in a year and then five years' time. This is how I came up with the idea of Tanya Burr Cosmetics and have continued to grow the brand. I want to make sure it always stays strong.

NOTES

List the things you would like to accomplish…

- -

- -

- -

- -

- -

- -

- -

- -

- -

- -

- -

- -

- -

- -

- -

- -

♡

NOTES

List your dream jobs...

♡

NOTES

A bit of extra space for your ideas and scribbles...

♡

MY TOP 10
BOOKS

I Know Why the Caged Bird Sings by Maya Angelou

A Thousand Splendid Suns by Khaled Hosseini

The Night Circus by Erin Morgenstern

Harry Potter series by J. K. Rowling
(No specific one, I love them all!)

The English Patient by Michael Ondaatje

Little Women by Louisa May Alcott

The Ocean at the End of the Lane by Neil Gaiman

The Other Boleyn Girl by Philippa Gregory

Atonement by Ian McEwan

The Picture of Dorian Gray by Oscar Wilde

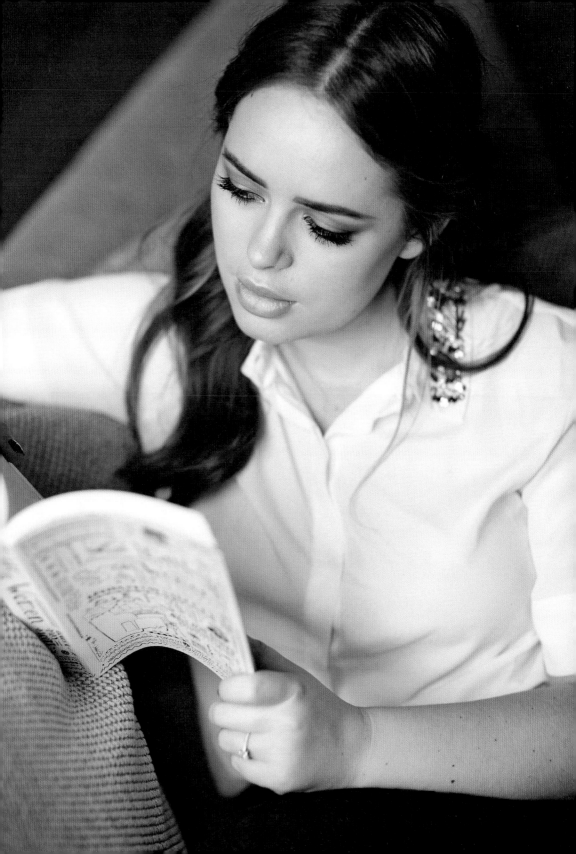

NOTES

List your favourite books here...

♡

ASK TANYA

Erin (@endlxssirwin)
Q: What was your favourite childhood tradition that you still do today?
A: Every New Year's Day, we go for a beach walk with my family and grandparents at Southwold in Suffolk. Even if I'm out really late the night before or it's freezing cold, we still go; Mum and Dad say it blows out the cobwebs at the start of the year.

Kayleigh (@kayleigh_ac)
Q: If you were a Disney character who would you be and why?
A: I'd be a mixture of Belle from *Beauty and the Beast* because she loves to read and sing, Tigger from *Winnie The Pooh* because he is bouncy and a bit excitable, and also Alice from *Alice in Wonderland* because she's a real dreamer.

Mikkeline (@mikkelinesm)
Q: How should I deal with schoolwork? I've got so much to do I can't possibly fit it all in my day?
A: Make a list of everything you need to do and tick it off as you go – if I have a long list of things to do, this always makes me feel so much better. Try and use your time wisely and prioritise the most important things and do them first. Good luck!

Corrie (@22corrie)
Q: What would your job be if you weren't a blogger?
A: When I was little I wanted to drive an ice cream van but now I'd quite like to have a cake shop and bake all the cakes myself!

Luella (@luellaworrow)
Q: How should I deal with rumours that aren't true?
A: The best thing to do, however hard it might be, is to ignore them. The people closest to you will know the truth.

Jessica (@tanyaburr_x)
Q: What are five things you should always have on you?
A: Money, your phone, your keys, lip balm and a smile!

Becky (@beckythellama)
Q: What's your favourite ice cream flavour?
A: I can't choose between mint choc chip and salted caramel – just not together!

Torrie (@_torrieholder_)
Q: What inspired you to keep going and never give up?
A: My passion for what I am doing, belief in myself, and the people watching my videos and reading my blog who encouraged me to keep going.

Rachel (@oakleysmd)

Q: If you could relive one moment in your entire life, what would it be?

A: When Jim proposed to me because it was such a blur of happiness and was over so quickly, so I'd love to do it again.

Jemima (@jemxx_)

Q: What inspires your videos?

A: It depends on what kind of video I'm making. It could be anything from a request someone has tweeted me, seeing a beauty or fashion campaign while walking past a shop window or just a random idea that has popped into my head.

ACKNOWLEDGEMENTS

Many, many thanks are due here:

To my managers, Dom and Lucy, at Gleam who have worked incredibly hard to help me realise my dreams.

To the wonderful people at Penguin, Fenella Bates and Emma Young, for such a warm welcome into the world of books and remarkable teamwork.

To Georgina Rodgers, for helping me to write my first book.

To the amazing creative team, Dan Kennedy, Matt Russell, Smith & Gilmour, Annie Swain, Samantha Cusick and Kolbrun Ran.

To all the lovely people who watch my videos, read my blog and chat to me on Twitter for their constant support and enthusiasm, which has guided and will continue to guide me through this adventure.

To my friends for their unstinting advice with everything I do and for always being there for me at the drop of a hat.

But most of all, as ever, to my family and Jim, thank you for believing in me from the beginning and giving me the strength and encouragement I needed to be the best I can be. From little dreams to sky-is-the-limit dreams, thank you for allowing me to live mine.